Humble Pie

Humble Pie

Sober Menopause, Sugar Addiction, and the Sweetness of Recovery

Dana Bowman

BLOOMSBURY ACADEMIC
NEW YORK • LONDON • OXFORD • NEW DELHI • SYDNEY

BLOOMSBURY ACADEMIC

Bloomsbury Publishing Inc, 1359 Broadway, New York, NY 10018, USA
Bloomsbury Publishing Plc, 50 Bedford Square, London, WC1B 3DP, UK
Bloomsbury Publishing Ireland, 29 Earlsfort Terrace, Dublin 2, D02 AY28, Ireland

BLOOMSBURY, BLOOMSBURY ACADEMIC and the Diana logo are trademarks of
Bloomsbury Publishing Plc

First published in the United States of America 2026

Copyright © Dana R. Bowman, 2026

Cover design by Diana Nuhn
Cover image front © iStock.com/Say-Cheese; back © iStock.com/Strawberry Blossom;
© iStock.com/Inkanya Anankitrojana

All rights reserved. No part of this publication may be: i) reproduced or transmitted in any form, electronic or mechanical, including photocopying, recording or by means of any information storage or retrieval system without prior permission in writing from the publishers; or ii) used or reproduced in any way for the training, development or operation of artificial intelligence (AI) technologies, including generative AI technologies. The rights holders expressly reserve this publication from the text and data mining exception as per Article 4(3) of the Digital Single Market Directive (EU) 2019/790.

Bloomsbury Publishing Inc does not have any control over, or responsibility for, any third-party websites referred to or in this book. All internet addresses given in this book were correct at the time of going to press. The author and publisher regret any inconvenience caused if addresses have changed or sites have ceased to exist, but can accept no responsibility for any such changes.

Library of Congress Cataloging-in-Publication Data
Names: Bowman, Dana author
Title: Humble pie : sober menopause, sugar addiction, and the sweetness of recovery / Dana Bowman.
Description: New York : Bloomsbury Academic, 2026. | Includes index. |
Identifiers: LCCN 2025024750 (print) | LCCN 2025024751 (ebook) |
ISBN 9798881800819 hardback | ISBN 9798881800826 epub |
ISBN 9798765160367 adobe pdf
Subjects: LCSH: Bowman, Dana | Recovering alcoholics--United States--Biography | Addicts--United States--Biography | Middle-aged women--United States--Biography | LCGFT: Autobiographies
Classification: LCC HV5137 .B6924 2026 (print) | LCC HV5137 (ebook) |
DDC 362.292092 [B]--dc23/eng/20250725
LC record available at https://lccn.loc.gov/2025024750
LC ebook record available at https://lccn.loc.gov/2025024751

ISBN: HB: 979-8-8818-0081-9
ePDF: 979-8-7651-6036-7
eBook: 979-8-8818-0082-6

Typeset by Deanta Global Publishing Services, Chennai, India
Printed and bound in the United States of America

For product safety related questions contact productsafety@bloomsbury.com.

To find out more about our authors and books visit www.bloomsbury.com and sign up for our newsletters.

*To Brian. You are in this book a lot. I love you.
And to the League of Good Women, of course.*

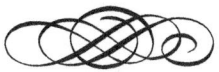

Contents

Introduction 1

Part I Addiction and Menopause

1   Thirst 7
2   Isolation 23
3   I'm Hungry 45
4   I'm Hungry: The Sequel 57
5   Vacancy 69
6   Risk 83

Part II Recovery

7   Marriage Is What Brings Us Together Today 99
8   The League of Good Women 109
9   Veggie Rehab 125
10 I Don't Want to Talk About It 137
11 Parenting Is Impossible 139

Part III Dessert

12 Stand Up 159
13 Forgiveness and Permission 179
14 Foreverness 197
15 Change 209

16 Flow 223
17 Are You Any Fun? 239
18 Big Time Dessert 255

Epilogue: Hashtag Blessed 259
A Recipe for Lemon Pie 261
Index 263
About the Author 265

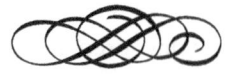

Introduction

Soon her eye fell on a little glass box that was lying under the table: she opened it, and found in it a very small cake, on which the words "EAT ME" were beautifully marked in currants. "Well, I'll eat it," said Alice, "and if it makes me grow larger, I can reach the key; and if it makes me grow smaller, I can creep under the door; so either way I'll get into the garden, and I don't care which happens!"

ALICE'S ADVENTURES IN WONDERLAND BY LEWIS CARROLL

Lemon pie, if done right, should hurt just a little.

When you eat a slice of lemon pie, the tartness should make your tongue and your brain do a tiny wince, but then the cloud of meringue melts it away. The slice needs to be ice cold and paired with a cup of very hot black coffee, which is served in a thick white mug. This is the pie I had in a small diner in North Carolina, and it made me want to cry.

Humble Pie will be about my long-term sobriety. It starts in a diner in North Carolina, as all good books should, and it takes me through mental health challenges, a global pandemic, nutball hormones, menopause, and physical illness, all while staying sober. It's like my very own telenovela, but without the spray tans and sleeping around.

My recovery is everything. It is the music in my life, my soundtrack that keeps me grooving forward, no matter the chaos around me. It's what wakes me up, and it's what lays me down.

But in that diner, with my slice of lemon pie, I could no longer hear the music. The pie was so *good*. But I devoured it in seconds. I stared at the crumbs on my plate, and I was still so hungry.

I wanted *more*.

Here is what I knew at the time: I knew that the waitress could bring endless slices of pie. She could keep marching in, slinging plates down, like those aggressive brooms in *The Sorcerer's Apprentice*, with all their sloshing pails of water overflowing the cauldron. I would never feel full.

My slice of lemon pie and I were on my tour for my second book, *How to Be Perfect Like Me*.[1] For those of you who don't know, a book tour is when people stand in front of you with your book in their hands and then want to talk about it. This is wonderful and terrifying at the same time, which is pretty much how all writing goes. Some folks will grill you over specific events in the book that you forgot you wrote. Others will say things like, "You are too funny about sobriety; this is serious," and then walk away. This surprises you so much that you laugh but then try to stifle it, and then you end up issuing a weird snuffle at the next guy.

People assume book tours are super glamorous, and they can be if you are Brene Brown. As an indie book author, however, my book tour had moments of true joy, but it also had stops where only two people showed up to my signing, and they were the store owner's parents. Weirdly, this happened twice on this trip. Shout-out to the parents for being so supportive. Meanwhile, each leg of my journey was becoming the Tour de Cinnamon Roll. I was anxious and tired and trying to celebrate my second book, but instead, all I wanted was pastry and a dark place to eat it.

I knew I was veering away from my sober path, into the land of food addiction and binge-eating, but I couldn't stop. Menopause, food addiction's bitchy sister, had swerved me into deep weeds. I am menopausal, therefore, I am invisible. Or at least it felt that way.

Months later, the isolation and fear of a global pandemic entered this hormonal mix of misery, and I succumbed to more unhealthy issues with comparison, scrolling, and frenetic over-exercising to compensate.

Finally, about a year later, my higher power threw up his hands and said, "Ok. You are a mess. It's time to deal." So I started writing about it all.

Humble Pie is in three parts. The first portion (Addiction and Menopause) describes the sneaky strength of behavioral addictions. Behavioral addictions, also called process addictions, are non-substance addictions. They are a set of behaviors, like gambling or shopping, that snare us. I have presented on this topic at various conferences, and so many women have approached me and reiterated that some of these behavioral addictions hunkered down and waited around until their sober selves were feeling pretty confident about their release from alcohol. Then, these addictions showed up, all excited to star in the second act. My audience members would lean into me and sigh, "I had no idea how hard this would be to stop. I thought I fully understood 'stopping' after I gave up drinking . . . but I'm so *stuck*."

Part II (Recovery) discusses how my recovery did some heavy lifting during this second act. In my early days of sobriety, I remember asking wistfully at a recovery meeting, "So . . . I think it's not actually about the wine . . . right?" and everyone just kind of chuckled. I found this completely annoying. And yet, here we are.

Humble Pie is a reckoning experience. It's about tussling with a daily acceptance practice about aging. Going gray and battling a difficult hearing diagnosis does not mean that I am a non-person, or that I no longer have anything to contribute to this world, but there are times when my addictions like to tell me otherwise. *Humble Pie* is also about finally naming my fixation on certainty, and how *waves hands around* all this, the relentless *lifeyness* of life cannot be bothered with the concept. And, *Humble Pie* is about admitting that hiding wads of Snickers wrappers under my mattress after a binge is very much like years before when I had stashed empty vodka bottles in my closet.

In early recovery, indulging in all the Snickers was necessary, and there was no shame. I needed the sugar. But in my last binge, while I was scarfing through a bag of fun-size Milky Ways,[2] and wrappers were fluttering around me like guilty confetti, I tried to tell myself, "Well, it's not vodka from my closet, so this is okay." But it wasn't anymore. I had to face that I was addicted to impulsive behaviors and also to drama-diving, and that meant not being over-dramatic about it all.

Part III (Dessert) is about the sweetness of recovery. I address the idea that "forever" is the forest through the recovery trees. I wrestle with annoying terms like "mom-guilt" and "balance." And, there's cleanup. There's always cleanup, especially in terms of relationships. Sobriety is just a continuing opening of dusty rooms to be aired out and set right. My oldest son is now sixteen. And, did you know? Teenagers *fray* things. It's part of their job description. Parenting my boys through the fear of "What if they become like me?" is tough. Fear made me threadbare. But finally, my soul mustered up some courage to say to me, "Excuse me, Miss? Your addictions are showing."

Behavioral addictions can shine a harsh light right through the fabric of our recovery. This is a good thing. We need light to recover.

Notes

1 A sweet little old lady once asked me what my book was called, and I told her. And she stood there, pursed her lips, and eyed me. I added, "It's ironic." She responded, "Oh. I see" in a way that indicated she did not. I slunk away.

2 I don't even *like* Milky Ways. Eating them is like when you bring home a giant bag of off-brand Fruit Spinsies from the bottom shelf of the cereal aisle to your boys. They taste of disappointment.

Part I

Addiction and Menopause

1

Thirst

A newly sober friend texted me one night. It was 9 p.m., so it was extremely late.

I can't do this. It's too hard. I can't do sober

She's right. "Doing" sobriety is a challenge. It's more like a "be." Let's try being. Being in our skin. Being still. Being with others and being with ourselves, even if both parties can occasionally be lousy company.

Being ok with not being ok.

Did I text all that to my friend? No. Too many words. I told her to take off her bra and her pants and get into bed. It's difficult to drive to the liquor store without pants. I've done it without a bra many times, but no pants is a force field.

I finished with this:

stay under the covers till morning

In the whole first year of sobriety, covers served me well.

I had a big green parka that made me look like a walking recycling bin. Its hood was expansive and furry and covered nearly all of my face. My parka and I went to the grocery store and the library. We attended church together. When I removed it, I felt naked and irritable, so I would put it back on. Sometimes I would sit in church pews or at band concerts, with the parka scooting up my neck and covering my ears and chin with fur and impenetrability. I had a scarf too, large, plaid, and orange, and I would wrap it over my nose. Because of scarf, I didn't have to talk to anyone. This scarf rule was my own, and I am sure folks tried to converse with me, but I replied with a short crinkle of my eyes to tell them I am a nice person, but I had on a scarf. The woolly warmth of it kept my words close. I saved my words for meetings and prayers. That's about it.

I traveled to my counselor and recovery meetings under the cover of night and scarf. Otherwise, it was me, my couch, a blanket, and a whole bunch of carbs. My body became covered in an extra layer of smoosh. I ate a lot of sugar, and that was fine. I *smooshed*.

I had become something soft and fuzzy and burrowed into things. This included my husband, who is also large and rather fuzzy. I clung to him like an alcoholic possum. He often saved the day for me and the kids when I would text him things like this:

Can u cook dinner?

No explanation. No real excuse. I just . . . couldn't. Newly sober Dana found the world full of sharp edges. Bumping up against another meal preparation without a gin and tonic in my hand felt impossible. Brian didn't ask about this. I honestly don't know if he had accepted that I was going to be the absolute worst from here on, but he didn't inquire.[1] He would just come home and make burgers, and the kids acted like it was the best thing ever while I covered up with another blanket and watched polite people make Victorian sponges on *The Great British Bake Off*. My sons would come in and crawl under the covers too, because Mom was so smooshy and soft. We would lie there, watching the Victorian sponge, and I would think, "I should make one of those," and then promptly forget about it.[2]

My central nervous system had been hijacked by alcohol for over twenty years. I had some healing to do.

The concept of hibernation has been researched quite a bit, and yet it still manages to mystify scientists. As I am a sucker for a good rodent article, I found out about an animal called the Arctic ground squirrel, which looks like a chillier version of every other ground squirrel you have ever seen. But these little rodents stand out in one very cool way. When they awake from seven months of sleeping and finally come snuffling out of their homes, their brains kind of *bloom*. After a nap, they don't yawn groggily and mutter "Don't talk to me I need coffee," and then sit in the recliner and stare into space for an hour to boot up. Nope. Rapidly, just within hours of waking, their squirrel brains start to regenerate and strengthen neural pathways, which demonstrates amazing brain plasticity. After hibernation, Arctic ground squirrels roll out and go hard, right into brain surge. The nap leads to squirrel growth. *Fast* growth.

And this is kind of what happened to me (yes, I'm the squirrel here), in recovery. In the first few months of sobriety, I hibernated. I hunkered down. I stored up for winter. I rested. Every once in a while, I would peek out of my hole and then shake my head "No" and lumber back into sleep.

And then, I woke up. At some point, I woke up, and I bloomed all over the place.[3] It was a miracle. I started running again (not from things, just as a workout). I cooked dinner again. I started to really laugh again. I wrote two books. TWO. I had dreamt of becoming an author since I was four years old.

I found my place in the world as a sober woman.

But because life is a journey and it's hard and because I am who I am, there is more to tell. Don't you, dear reader, ever get tired of hearing how life is a journey and it's hard? I do. I once told a friend of mine that I didn't like working on myself all the time, to which she shot back, "What, like it's hard?"

That second book, *How to Be Perfect Like Me*, was about my relapse.[4] Writing it was about as fun as the relapse itself, but I have to admit I was looking forward to its book tour because a book tour means you have Made It as a Big Author. You are basically signing autographs because you're famous, at least in the niche of alcoholic writers. I'll take my cool wherever I can. But, one of the side effects of book tours is talking to a lot of strangers, and this was *not* cool, in my opinion. I don't know how I hadn't anticipated this. Perhaps I was planning on doing the tour with my green parka?

A book tour was a new thing. And since I was doing something new, my expectations were dialed up to high filtration, like those glowy glamour shot pictures from the 1980s, where you placed your hand on your chin in a way that no one ever did in the history of gestures. My book tour had a *glow* to it.

In reality, of course, the book tour was just a book tour. It meant a different hotel every two nights and showing up to bookstores with one hopeful bookstore manager, a lot of chairs set up in neat rows, and a ticking clock. The bookstore manager and I would eye the clock, both trying not to mention that only three of the chairs were filled and the event was due to start in two minutes. This was not easy on my anxious heart.

My first leg of the book tour was hosted by a large library in Des Moines, where I would be giving a talk about my sober journey and then signing books. On the first night, I walked up to the community center where it would be held, and I noticed all the usual suspects. There were signs for chair yoga on the entrance doors. A sweet woman in a flowy linen dress was setting up a large pile of my books for signing, right next to a cool water feature that trickled and made me look around for a bathroom. As I entered the space, I saw my podium and a microphone that no one really knew how to work, and lots of seats.

And nobody is yet *in* the seats. No. One.

Finally, about fifteen people arrived, but I thought I might have a mild anxiety attack before, during, and after. I went into the bathroom at least twice to reapply lipstick and stare into the mirror. A tired woman with new wrinkles on her neck stared back. I wondered where the exits were.

I called my husband. He didn't pick up, and I texted:

Why am I doing this again?

He texted back:

Sorry I can't respond right now; I am driving in Focus and I am unable to answer the call.

I checked my hair in the mirror, lifted my mouth into a smile, and did the next right thing, which meant leaving the bathroom.

Sparsely attended signings were not the case for the entire trip. I did have events that involved people. But that first gathering felt so small, and that smallness held onto me. I felt embarrassed for the library that was holding it. They had advertised, yes, but for some reason, folks didn't want to come sit and talk about addiction. I decided there were a couple of reasons for this:

1. Addiction book signings might massively point to the signee as the addict.
2. I am massively boring.

The term "imposter syndrome" was originally only attributed to women, which is a clueless way of saying, "Ohhh. Are you struggling with feeling inadequate at your workplace? That's just so YOU. So, get up on that mental health horse and fix it! You go, Mom Boss!" The reality is that in many cases, the workplace created those exclusionary hurdles for women in the first place. Telling a woman to stop feeling alienated in an alienating workplace is kind of like when I find a week-old bowl of ramen-cement under my son's bed, and then the culprit says, "Why you actin' all mad?"

Also, can we just stop calling it "imposter" anything? Women are not imposters, and we don't need another "other" label to manage right now. We are busy.

My feelings of inadequacy started talking to me a lot on this book tour. Before *Perfect*, I was just happy to be here, a writer, with an actual book. But with this tour and with my faltering confidence, a committee of Big Important Author People started forming in my head. And it told me: "Yeah, we know this is your second book, but we've decided we don't have a seat for you here. You didn't make the list."

Really? That's such a mean thing to say. I honestly don't think there are any authors out there who would be that mean in real life. Maybe there's one or two, but I think generally we are a likable bunch.

And I do grasp that there are some writer tables I won't sit with in this life. Probably not going to be at Brene Brown's table. That's ok. But I could still be in the room, Brene Brown *adjacent*, if you will, so I could maybe wave across the tables to her in an awkward way. But the awful committee in my head was stopping me at the door and saying, "There is NO table here for you, Dana. Not even a small one over with the kids. *Why did you ever think you could show up here at all?*"

As a result, a sort of motion-sickness progression began. I seemed to dip into procrastination on this trip, putting off tweaking my speaking script, pushing off any sort of work on a new book or writing deadlines, dropping into daily malaise with a sickening swoop, like I was on a rickety coaster at a county fair. Then, at a well-attended event, I would slowly climb to the heights as I would speak about my book to a crowd. I would crest on good feelings, only to plummet later that evening, fueled by my overthinking. "You're just lucky! Wheeeeeee!" my insecurity would scream as I ricocheted around on the ride. "This isn't reeeeeaaallllll!"

One of my stops on the tour was in a lovely bookstore in Omaha, Nebraska. It was the kind of place with nooks and crannies, a coffee bar, and lots of cozy chairs tucked away in corners. There were bookmarks with cats dressed up in Victorian clothes. It felt like what a rom-com would establish as Quaint Bookstore Where They Fall In Love.

I showed up late because traffic in Omaha is intense. I didn't expect this, as perhaps most of us wouldn't, and I was unable to find a place to park. So, when I finally entered the front door and was ushered back to the location of the podium, my heart sank. I saw an elderly couple in the front row, waiting for me. Only two.

This was my nightmare.

This was the lowest number I had experienced on this trip. But I plastered on a smile, set my copy of my book on the podium, and proceeded to talk directly to these two about my life for twenty minutes. I finished up, thanked them for coming, and the manager gestured gamely to my table, where I would perhaps sign two books for two people.

One of the two approached me. She said, "Thank you for your lovely talk. We're not going to get a book, though. We're here for our son. He owns the bookstore."

I looked over at the manager. He sighed and shrugged. I smiled and shrugged. And something inside of me crumpled.

This would be the event I would hold onto when people asked me about the book tour. "Oh! A book tour!" my friends would say. "That sounds so cool!" and I would chuckle and take out this story to share with them. I would polish my self-effacement to a brilliant shine.

But I wouldn't *really* talk about it. Not even to my husband. Not even to myself. Because I couldn't put it into words, this tiny, colossal thing. The insecurity festered quietly. It had advanced well past chiding me that my skills were lacking, that I wasn't a good writer. Now, it simply said to me, "You are not worth it." And for some reason, I listened.

In my early twenties, I attended a summer writing program affiliated with the prestigious Iowa Writers Workshop at the University of Iowa. This was back when I was single, wore flannel, and wrote poetry a lot. I was *earnest*. My instructor at the workshop told me I had talent, and I believed him.[5] I knew I had talent. I knew I could write. I soaked up the classes and bookishness like an earnest, writerly sponge. I had a list of *New Yorker* editors' addresses on a piece of paper. I was ready. I was going to be a writer.

Each day during the workshop, Iowa City's glorious bookstore, Prairie Lights, would host reading events called Elevenses. "Elevenses" sounds just a teensy bit pretentious, and also like something a hobbit would do. Second breakfast? Sure. Let's have *elevenses*. As I was a slightly pretentious twenty-year-old but also a total LOTR geek, I attended nearly all of them. As I sat there, rapt, listening to an author talk about her new literary novel, I studied her. She had draped herself in a large red scarf, and her hair surrounded her face in a dark cloud. She had a tinkly bracelet that percussed her thoughts. The next day, I wore bracelets and wore my hair down. And I soaked it all in. This writing thing. It felt like red lipstick, like possibility.

One day, I thought. *One day, I might be at that podium.*

The thought was so precious and bright that it shone like a tiny diamond.

So after *How to Be Perfect* had been published, and I entered Prairie Lights bookstore for my own book reading during my book tour, I felt it. I did. I opened the jewel box of a dream from long ago, and I stared at it. And then I gave a talk about my book to a packed house. This was no imposter situation. This was real and lovely, and as I walked to my car afterward, I remembered thinking, *This is exactly right.*

So, why didn't that experience cancel out the empty chairs at some of the other events? Why don't I always go back to Prairie Lights as my beacon? Why, instead, do I remember the two parents of the bookseller? Or the woman who loudly asked me at one book reading, "Are you funny? Can you read some funny parts?" as if my humor was some sort of funny, sober rabbit I could pull out of a hat?

Why do I focus on the bad stuff so much more than the good?

Other Bad Things I Remember with Amazing Clarity

1. When I was in seventh grade, I was on the drill team, and we had a pool party. I was the only one who wore a one-piece suit. Awful.

2. Once, when I was shopping at Big Crowded Overwhelming Bulk Store, I didn't maneuver my cart around this old man who was approaching me, and he sneered, "Excuse YOU," really loudly to me, and I was so shocked by his rudeness that I wasn't able to come up with a good comeback. This was nearly four years ago. I still think about him.

3. I had a seventh-grade choir concert during school, and I wore my choir dress in the morning and forgot to bring a change of clothes. After the performance, I hid in the gym locker room because my mom was unable to bring clothes. I stayed there until fifth hour when I finally attended social studies in my blue polyester floor-length dress because I was too afraid I would get in trouble with Mr. Staed. That day was mortification with a fear chaser.

4. In my twenties, a boyfriend once used the phrase "rounded shoulders" with me, and since then, I have always been convinced I have a mild Quasimodo vibe going on.

These moments (and they were just moments, even if Mr. Staed's social studies class seemed like an eternity) glare at me. Highly colorized and over-saturated, I take them out every once in a while and turn them around in my mind, just to make sure they still hurt. They don't disappoint—the sharp sting of realizing my swimsuit was causing the girls to snicker while one girl, Laura Sinclair, loudly laughed, "Oh Dana! Look at *you*!" was devastating. It was at that point in my seventh-grade life that I grasped how massively important it was to wear a hot pink Body Glove bikini to the pool, but my mom wouldn't allow me to wear a two-piece yet. Before that, what I wore on my body was just . . . what I wore on my body. When I caught a glimpse of myself in the pool's warped bathroom mirror, I suddenly realized: I was wearing a one-piece *with ruffles*. I was doomed.

I have two dogs, Rey and Hosmer, and when I am a good dog owner, I take them on walks. Rey is large and blonde and fluffy. She is . . . big. Big-boned. Gorgeous. She's a healthy Swedish milkmaid dog with a large smile and capable paws. Hosmer is small and wiry and always looks like he thinks he's about to be mugged. On one walk, Rey suddenly started limping, head down, face sad. Her whole blond body seemed to curl up in pain. "Ohhh! My darling! What is it?" I said as I knelt in front of her. I think she realized this was her moment because she flopped down on her side, curled around the offending paw with such a look of grief that I nearly burst into tears for her. I gently cradled the paw and cooed at Rey, convinced she'd been mortally wounded. She lolled her head down on the sidewalk and *looked* mortally wounded. Hosmer grunted and sat down. He rolled his eyes.

It was a burr, about the size of a bit of rice, stuck between her toe pads. It was tiny, and I flicked it away and eyed her. She groaned and stretched out on the sidewalk, enjoying the warmth of the concrete, and that we all just about attended her funeral about two minutes ago. Hosmer tugged at the leash and checked his watch. That tiny burr had all but maimed my precious, and even when she got up to walk the rest of the way home, we took it easy. It was traumatic.

That teensy tiny burr took my behemoth of a dog *out*. My tiny, spiky moments of negativity do too. I limp along and stop and scout them out, then hold them up and squint at them in the light. Tiny but terrible little memories stick with me and make me limp along. I analyze the empty chairs at the bookstore, or that one negative review on Goodreads,[6] or the memory of how hard it was to write certain chapters of my books, or the endless slights and errors that occur when you are working on something really important to you.

This sort of makes sense. Negative experiences involve more thinking than positive ones. It's called "negativity bias." Negativity is just . . . chewier. For example, when people describe bad events, they use stronger words to explain the incident. And some statistics say up to 80 percent of our thoughts are negative, which is a gloomy thought in itself, and I now invite you to join me in an endless loop of thinky awfulness. In my recovery group, we have a saying[7] for this: "First thought wrong." But in my case, it isn't just the first thought that was awry. It's the second, the third . . . It's a whole parade of wrong.

I invest in negative thoughts, but the good ones just glide on by. The last time I got an ice cream cone from our little town's ice cream shop, I didn't take a lick and then immediately analyze why I was enjoying it so much. My sons, who tagged along because they're fulfilling the "endless mooch" part of their contracts, walked home with me as we ate our dripping cones, and I'm not thinking, "Hm. It's weird how much of a good time we're having here. I wonder why I am so pleased by this ice cream/son ratio. What does it all *mean*?" Happiness over a cone of deliciously tart key lime ice cream doesn't have much subtext.

Perhaps that makes happiness shallow, but I don't think she minds because she is too busy enjoying herself.

Interestingly, an infiltration of negativity surfaces once I've finished the cone. These thoughts show up late, but like that one kid who only worsens his tardiness by shouting "WHATSUP MY DUDES" as he slams through the door, they get a lot of attention. I start to wonder about the calories in my ice cream cone, and why I didn't try to power-walk home. I'll contemplate a salad for dinner, and then I'll mull over how I kind of hate salad. I'll spend an inordinate amount of time just thinking about how fat-free dressing makes me angry. And so on.

In the 1990s I was hired for my first teaching job. I was so stoked about this that I also accepted a position as the school's theater producer, even though I had no clue how to do this. I just signed my contract and then spent the next year embracing the scrappy, "Hey! Let's put on a show!" vibe of those Little Rascals kids.

I chose *You're a Good Man, Charlie Brown* as my first musical because it had minimal sets and the songs were kidlike, so we could fake talent. One of the main characters was a dog, ok? It was going to be alright. I had no idea how to run lighting, so I found a senior who was in honors classes and handed him the instruction manual for the light board. "I'm sure you can figure this out," I told him, "I'll just be over here doing choreography that I am pulling out of thin air, but one of our main characters is a dog. It's going to be alright."

And surprisingly, it was. The dog got a standing ovation (shout out to Trey Miller, who is probably the CEO of something now). At no point during all this do I remember thinking, "What if I can't do this?" I just . . . *did* it. Sure, the doghouse would sway a bit when Trey had to climb it for his solo number, but that just embellishes the tension of the scene.[8]

Why didn't insecurity make an entrance when Lucy missed her cues because she was flirting backstage with Linus, which is just so very wrong? Or when our mics stuttered so much that the audience probably only heard 75 percent of the show? Perhaps it was youthful ignorance and energy. Or that I was drinking back then. It was probably some combination of both. I was twenty-five and clueless, with less time to stir up the negative thought patterns that had solidified into congealed blocks of unease in my fifties. Oh, the blessed lightness of youth.

With time, there are more memories. It's science. We get older, and we get more stuff. There is a tricky part about getting older—it tells you that you should have it all together because of wisdom, but in my case, I think it just means I've had more time to percolate. My brain, which is the alcoholic kind, stirred my memories into a special sauce. Studies have shown that alcoholics do tend to worry more than normies. And from worry, these thoughts brewed right into rumination. From there? I had arrived at an emotional disorder psychiatrists call Repeated Negative Thinking (RNT), which is a boring label for something so powerful. I think RNT lacks a snazzy title, like: This One Thing from 2002 Is Going to Mess You Up *for Ten Years*.

Alcoholics are more prone to RNT. So are women. And, I bet you guessed it, so are perfectionists. Basically, I didn't have much of a chance of making it out of the RNT zone in one piece, but I sure wish I had known sooner that it was a diagnosable thing, with its boring but useful name. It's nice to have a label for things sometimes. As my mom put it, way back when I was about ten years old, "Dana, you tend to mull over things." I'm a muller. It's true. For the longest time, I was able to throw a party for me and my mulls, and we'd all settle down for a bit. They'd be muttering and getting into my business, and I'd say, "Hey! Let's have some vodka!" and then they'd leave me alone.

But damn if I didn't get sober and have to deal with life on life's terms.

And damn if now, some four years later, life and all its incessant lifey-ness were messing with me.[9]

My book tour and I were having a hard time.

What happened next was a bit of a wake-up call. I wrecked my rental car, and all I could think about was a box of cupcakes.

So first of all, I blame some of this on the Kia Sportage (which, in my head, I always referred to as the Sport-*ahhhgge*). This car and I did not like each other much. It tried to be sporty, but it was seriously uncool. When I was about three miles away from the rental place, it started making a strange thwacking noise whenever I made a left turn. This made all future left turns nerve-wracking. The thwacking did mysteriously stop after ten miles or so, but it was sealed: this car, as my kids would call it, was a "sus." And yes, I should have turned around and taken it back to the rental place, but I have always been the sort of "let's just see and wait it out" kind of person, and I just realized that explains why I became an alcoholic. Also, returning to the rental place would have merited another left turn, and we were avoiding those.

Additionally, the back windows of my Sportahhhgge were just there for show. They were tiny and weirdly placed, and there was no way you were going to get visuals on them.

On the last day of my trip, on my way to my hotel, I made a wrong turn.[10] I needed to back out and head down the road a bit more. It was raining, and my GPS had also been sus for all of this trip, and I had just finished my final speaking event. I was in that weird tired-elated place because the day had been amazing. The audience had been enthusiastic, and I received an actual standing ovation. Also, the luncheon following featured barbecue, so maybe that's what the applause was all about. I didn't care. The whole thing had been wonderful. So, when I made the wrong turn, I was distracted, tired, and also couldn't see. This wreck was completely *not* my fault.

I reversed onto the road, right into an oncoming car, coming at me at about forty miles an hour.

It was *so* my fault.

As far as wrecks go, it could have been worse. The woman who was the victim of my driving was not injured, and she actually managed to soothe *me* about running into *her*.[11] She was nice. The police officer who had to deal with all of this was also really nice. I would like to say the people from the rental company were nice as well, but I don't know. I talked to about fourteen of them on the phone, so it got confusing. I have never really been a customer service kind of girl (this goes right along with my let's wait and see policy about life), and so the phone calls were tough.

I was exhausted. Meanwhile, something weird was happening in my brain. The police officer and the insurance people kept asking me questions about VINs and policy numbers and insurance agent numbers, and I was doing this floaty thing where all I could think about was the six cupcakes in a cute pink box in the back of the Sportahhhgge. At one point, I ran out to the car, which I had parked at the entrance of the hotel, and peered in the tiny back windows. It was pouring rain, and I had told the policeman that I needed to check if I had left anything else in the back seat, but honestly? I wanted to make sure my cupcakes were all right. It was all I could think about. Cupcakes.

It is embarrassing to admit, but all I wanted was to get to my hotel room so that I could eat these cupcakes. All six of them. After the book signing, I stopped off at a bakery on the way, needing something to help me "celebrate" the end of the tour. I don't drink anymore, right? So, when I saw a storefront with a colorful pink and white striped awning, I turned in. The front door opened with a cheerful bell, and the shop smelled like vanilla. I peered down at the rows of colorful frosting and carefully selected a nice variety: Chocolate mocha. Wedding cake. Lemon cream, of course. I bought a half dozen because I couldn't get just one; I knew that "just one" would only make me want more. I think I even said something to the girl waiting on me, "I'm going to have to share these!" and I told myself I would just eat a couple and save the rest for the next day.

I bought enough cupcakes so that I wouldn't have to fear running out. So that I would feel full. Full enough that I might sleep.

For the other alcoholics in the room, does any of this sound at all familiar?

Recovery is forever. It is stitched firmly into my daily life. Why? Because, for me, alcoholism is forever. I know this. I'm an alcoholic, and drinking is no longer a possibility for me. I learned this well after my first and final relapse and got sober one week later on New Year's Day. I KNOW this stuff. But I was starting to exhibit some addictive behaviors with food on this trip. My lemon pie in that diner had been a signal of this. I had found myself shoveling burgers, fries, and shakes at late-night chain restaurants more than once. At the airport, I bought overpriced packs of peanut M and M's and stashed them in my baggage. One night, I spent over fifty dollars on room service and mindlessly ate while watching *Say Yes to the Dress* episodes. I craved sugary coffee, sugary muffins, and sugary pastries for breakfast (I had always been a savory sort of breakfast person before). I just kept eating.

And now, all I wanted to do was close the door of my hotel room, lock it, change into some dry clothes, and eat those cupcakes. I *thirsted* for them.

About two hours later, when all the numbers in the world had been exchanged with the insurance people, I grabbed my purse and my slightly wilted pink box of cupcakes out of the car. I watched as the Kia was towed away in the rain. And then, I headed right to my room, shut the door with a sigh, and shut out the world. I clambered into bed with my box and a remote, pulled off the wrapper of the chocolate mocha, and ate it in four bites. I made it to cupcake number three before I slowed down. And I felt empty, the entire time.

And this is the pitiless experience of addiction. The more you shovel in, the less you have.

Notes

1. Honestly? Sometimes I wanted him to ask. I kind of wanted to *tussle* about this. I wanted him to come home and sigh heavily and say, "Are you going to EVER take off the parka? And by that, what I really mean is: Are you going to be the absolute worst, from here on?" And then I could burst into tears and tell him how hard this was (it was), and tell him he didn't understand (he didn't) and that he was an absolute asshole (very possibly). But he never asked. I think he had worked it out that if he DID ask, there would be a much larger asshole/not-asshole ratio going on here. Since he is an engineer, he just did the math in his head, kept quiet, and went outside to grill something. Sometimes that's the best thing you can do in a marriage. Keep quiet and go outside to grill something.

2. I did, in fact, make one of these cakes for my son's birthday this year. It was lopsided, and I used too much whipped cream, but can you ever really use too much whipped cream? I bedazzled it with fresh raspberries and then brought it forth, with fifteen candles, and when we sang Happy Birthday I tried out my British accent. I really mangled the accent, and then we mangled the cake, and this whole memory is a straight-up blessing of recovery.

3. I have heard repeatedly that "three" seems to be a physical and mental marker in addiction and recovery, and I think I agree. Three months sober, I started laughing again. Like, real, deep belly laughs. My husband once made me laugh so hard I started crying, which felt like a freaking miracle and also really confused him. At six months,

I really hit my stride, started writing, and started "blooming" more. I can remember attending meetings around this time and exclaiming how strong I felt in my recovery. So, if you're in the early days, think three. Three days. Three months. It will get better, and then it will get amazing.

4 Here's another interesting thing about the number three. I had been sober since 2011 when I relapsed three years later. I had been told to beware of big anniversaries, like one year, three years, that sort of thing. And in three years, I hit a block and relapsed while the Christmas holidays were in full swing. So, the number three came and bit me in the ass in this case. My relapse lasted one week, and it was straight hell. It also taught me a lot, but I don't recommend it to anyone, ever.

5 Tom Barbash. He is an excellent writer. After I signed my contract for *Bottled*, I sent him an email thanking him for his kindness to me during the conference. He didn't respond, but I'm sure he still thinks of me fondly from time to time. Ok probably not but I also have to admit that I signed up for his class mainly because he is totally handsome and pretty much fits the bill as "Hot Writer," so we're even.

6 One review said I was too positive, that I was the "Cinderella of sobriety." She meant it in a negative way, but I kind of think this review is the best thing ever.

7 We have a saying for everything.

8 I do realize that *You're a Good Man Charlie Brown* was not billed as a thriller. That's not really its vibe. As it was clearly felt from the beginning that pulling off this show would be a miracle, suspense was a creative choice.

9 Honestly, I would like to be able to write something like this: "Hey! I got sober and then my recovery and I were rock solid from there on. The end." But that would not be the truth. And recovery asks me to tell the truth. So here we are. But I will tell you that I have remained sober from alcohol since January 1, 2014. This book is about process addictions, but booze and I? We have been broken up for over ten years, and I am so grateful.

10 It was a right turn.

11 She was a physical therapist. She gave me a hug and said, "Hey, if I'm injured I can be my own PT." I bet she is a mom. We multitask. I am also forever grateful to her for her humor and kindness.

Bibiliography

1 **The concept of hibernation:**
Jabr, F. (2012, June 26). What the Supercool Arctic Ground Squirrel Teaches Us about the Brain's Resilience. *Scientific American*. https://www.scientificamerican.com/article/arctic-ground-squirrel-brain/.

2   . . . the workplace created exclusionary those hurdles for women:
Tulshyan, R., and J. A. Burey (2021, February 11). Stop Telling Women They Have Imposter Syndrome. *Harvard Business Review.* https://hbr.org/2021/02/stop-telling-women-they-have-imposter-syndrome.

3   **Negative experiences involve more thinking than positive ones:**
The Decision Lab. (2023). *Negativity Bias.* The Decision Lab. https://thedecisionlab.com/biases/negativity-bias.

4   . . . up to 80% of our thoughts are negative:
Johnson, C. (2023). *Stuck on Negative Thinking.* Care Counseling: Minnesota Therapists. https://care-clinics.com/stuck-on-negative-thinking/.

5   **My brain, which is the alcoholic kind, stirred my memories into a special sauce:**
Devynck, F., A. Rousseau, and L. Romo (2019, July 3). Does Repetitive Negative Thinking Influence Alcohol Use?. *A Systematic Review of the Literature. Frontiers in Psychology* 10: 1482. https://doi.org/10.3389/fpsyg.2019.01482.

6   **Alcoholics are more prone to RNT:**
Mollaahmetoglu, O. M., E. Palmer, and E. Maschauer, et al. (2021). The Acute Effects of Alcohol on State Rumination in the Laboratory. *Psychopharmacology* 238: 1671–86. https://doi.org/10.1007/s00213-021-05802-1.

7   **So are women:**
Johnson, D. P., and M. A. Whisman (2013, August). Gender Differences in Rumination: A Meta-Analysis. *Personality and Individual Differences* 55 (4): 367–74. https://doi.org/10.1016/j.paid.2013.03.019.

8   . . . so are perfectionists:
Sharp, Caitlin A. (2016). The Interaction Between Perfectionism and Rumination Predicting State Self-compassion. *Student Publications* 533. https://cupola.gettysburg.edu/student_scholarship/533.

2

Isolation

I don't watch scary movies anymore.

The last scary movie I watched was a "based on a true story" doozy called *The Exorcism of Emily Rose*. It was stressful. In the last half of the movie, I gripped onto my cat Steve for so long that he was really stressed out too, and he let me know by sinking his claws into my lap. So now I'm stressed **and** in pain.

Scary movies and I broke up for two reasons:

1. I get super invested in people's lives in movies and sad TV commercials. After I had kids, some sort of nervous empathy switch had been dialed up to eleven, and I'd be sitting watching *Independence Day* and muttering things like: "Oh all those people, and the aliens just flat out killed them. All of them. It's just so awful," while my boys would peel their eyes away from the explosions and say "You're being weird" just with their faces. This Emily Rose movie just made me so freaked out for Emily. She kept bending all the way backward, and that must have been painful.

2. I was sober when I watched this movie, so I was unable to coat its scariness with red wine.

Brian and I made it through, even with me asking stuff like, "Do you think she was able to make up all her work at school for her absences?" Then I went to bed and stared at the ceiling for about an hour, replaying the plot in my head. I wasn't scared, exactly. I think I took all my scared feelings and exchanged them for stress because I could manage that a bit more. I was just so *stressed out* about Emily Rose and her demon possession problem. There had to be so many strings attached. How was her mom? What was their insurance deductible for all this? Did they have to move? I would want to move. But that's a lot; moving is very stressful. And who would do all the packing? Would they have to clean that house before they left? Who would want to even deal with the scary room with all the upside-down crosses?

And so, that was my last scary movie. Turns out, this was a very wise choice because right around the same time, I had a speaking gig in Tucson. On the plane home, I read an article on my phone about a flu bug that was causing problems in Asia. "Weird," I thought. "That's too bad. I sure hope they'll be ok."

Who needs scary movies when life is scary enough?

By the end of 2022, 40 percent of us rated our stress levels as "fair to poor." The American Psychiatric Association reports that these numbers will only increase as a result of Covid-19. Go figure.

Because I like to be early, I had signed up for the "fair to poor" category back in 2020. Honestly, I think the spectrum from "fair" to "poor" is too wide. There needs to be an additional rating in the middle, something like: "Um. I'm ok today, I guess? I don't want to think about it." And the fallout continues. Bits of flak and apprehension flutter down around me at the grocery store or when I read the news. The other day, I saw a person with a mask on, a woman with short gray hair and glasses, and a fanny pack. She is small and looks like my mom. I wonder why she's wearing a mask. I wonder if she's angry at me for being here with her and **not** wearing a mask. I wonder at how angry we all are. That's a lot of thinking in the cereal aisle, but here we are. Ashes of distrust and accusations still float down all around us.

I worry about food prices and job losses. Buying produce feels like an indulgence, which is never how one should feel about buying kale. I found a bag of disposable face masks while I was cleaning out my car console, and my hand shrank back like it was a bag of spiders. I wanted to throw the whole pack away, and I saw myself one-handing it, tossing it in a heroic arc to swish into a nearby trash can. I would raise my hands in a little victory, hoping this act of riddance would just *solve* it.

But then a small voice said, "It could happen again," and I slammed the console shut. This voice is not buried deep; it's always bobbing around in the shallows. It says things like, "What if my parents get sick," and "We don't have any heroes anymore," and "The kids are messed up." Little statements of catastrophe float up like my brain is a Magic 8 ball of doom. They surface while I'm driving home, passing the school, watching the news, chopping expensive kale for dinner.

Basically, the vibe is doom, but also, I'm just so *busy*.

When I was twenty-eight, the man I thought I was going to marry decided he did not want to get married.[1] I think I knew for a good six months prior to the official breakup that this was going to happen, but I held onto that relationship with loyalty and stress, and while the whole thing was slowly grinding to a horrific halt, I bought a house.

The house was cute. Like, super cute. It was touted as a bungalow, which is real estate-speak for "This house has two closets." The living room was tiny, with the original fireplace that no longer worked and adorable shutters on all windows that fell apart if you touched them. I didn't care about any of these things because it was lovely and mine, and when Ryan finally broke it off, I decided to date my house. I decorated that house within an inch of its life. Everything was *just so*. And, I could set things down and they would stay there, unmoved, until I moved them again. This is a thing that I never realized would be a thing until after I had children. Children move things. And they never say, "Mother, this small ceramic turtle that you made when you were in third grade, that is lovingly placed here as decoration because it's whimsical? Well, I'm going to pocket it and put it in the upstairs bathtub where it will break, and I won't tell anyone about it until you try to take a shower, which will then turn into a first-aid shower. Ok?"

My sweet little bungalow became a Temple of Dana. I found two comfy indigo chairs at a garage sale and a bright Moroccan rug, and I festooned the room with white lights and old books. I bought cut flowers for myself every week and set them on my tiny antique table, where I was supposed to eat, but rarely did because my parents weren't around, so I just ate on the couch. The fireplace was shoved full of fat drippy candles, and it looked artistic and cool. I never dusted it or lit those candles, but it was perfect. My one bathroom had the original pink and black tile. Every inch of the space said Dana. I imprinted all over the thing. My house was an Instagram house before Instagram existed. And, there are times now, like when my husband buys a gray plastic digital weather station and installs it in the living room because it's super important to know the weather in there, that I just really miss my little bungalow.

I loved my house so much that I rarely left it. I would get up in the morning, get into my teacher uniform (khaki skirt, Gap cardigan, Steve Madden slides; it was the 1990s), and I would do the teacher show for nine hours. Then I would come home via the liquor store, and as soon as I entered the front door, a deep sigh would escape me. My college roommate once told me that she could hear that sigh from the foyer when I came home from classes. I am a sigh-er. There was something about reaching that front door that signified that I could be quiet again. I could lie down. I could relax. But at my little bungalow, this sigh signaled more. My face could slacken, and I didn't have to smile anymore. I didn't have to be *on*. I didn't owe anybody anything. And I would pour myself that beloved first glass of wine and take off my bra, and I felt like I had entered the Sky Lounge and I was the only member. Honestly, this still sounds kind of lovely, minus the wine. Nowadays, I come home and am immediately asked questions about snacks.

My bungalow and I continued hanging out. The best weekends were ones with movies and wine, and no people. Sometimes, late at night, I would go sit on my front stoop and feel a sharp needle of loneliness, but I figured the wine had only made me maudlin. I had my dog, Norman, a lot of cute stemware, and a freaking adorable house. The house understood me.

I didn't have to talk about heartbreak to anyone. I had tried, once, to tell a friend at work about my relationship that had ended. As I started to explain how I felt about Ryan, it felt like I was on a precipice, and my friend was just nodding at me. There was this impossible chasm between us, and trying to explain how deeply I loved him while she smiled at me just made me feel like walking off the edge. Talking made me feel more alone, which was kind of impossible since I had already been *left*. I didn't want to be alone-er.

So, I clammed up. Anguish simmered so close to the surface (pain does that; it longs to poke through the skin) that staying away from all the people seemed like the best solution.

My sister Jen is a breast cancer survivor. She once told me about a friend who spied her at the store and exclaimed to her, "I haven't seen you in so long! Where've ya been?" Jenni replied, kind of grimly, "I have been dealing with cancer." To which the friend took a beat and said, "Cancer! Cancer is such a bummer."

Jen told me, "A bummer? Cancer is a BUMMER? Like, really?"

Now, to be fair, the friend was probably just trying her best to respond in a way that was encouraging. And yes, cancer is a bummer. So is depression. It's a total bummer. So was the Titanic. But the chasm between her friends' words and how Jen felt? It added pain to pain. Which, it is true, is a total bummer.

So, you can either deal with people telling you that your cancer and mastectomy, and the ruthlessness of this disease, are a bummer, or you can hide away. Jen is an extrovert, so I'm pretty sure she did not do this. I, however, took my sadness and packaged it up into a small bungalow, and there I stayed.

I hid. And I drank. I worked through a lot of this when I got sober in 2014. I shone a light on the dark places that I had tucked away and started to acknowledge two truths about myself: I am an introvert, and it's ok to seek solace and sanctuary from people. But, maybe... It's also just plain old hiding.

Here's an infographic below to illustrate (Figure 2.1):

The hard part is realizing my gauge is almost always in the middle. It's tricky. If I'm leaning on the hiding side, though, things get even more complicated because then I have to get up, put on a bra, slink out from my hiding location, and do adult things I don't want to do. Which is, dare I say it? A bummer.

Isolation is very dangerous, especially for an alcoholic.

Cue: A global pandemic.

When I got the notification from our schools that they would be closing their doors and we would be learning at home, and the world was ending, I was at Target.

It's important to note that I have never much cared for shopping, but Target sure tries to make me like it. Shopping involves crowded aisles and this whole fake-smiling thing as you come around corners, and then we do that awkward "No, you go ahead" bit because we must hold onto social norms in this place. If humanity is going to fall apart, it's going to start at a grocery store, so I am always super polite in there to hold it off.

It's also important to note that the reason I was at Target was because I was on day two of a writing retreat. I had left home.

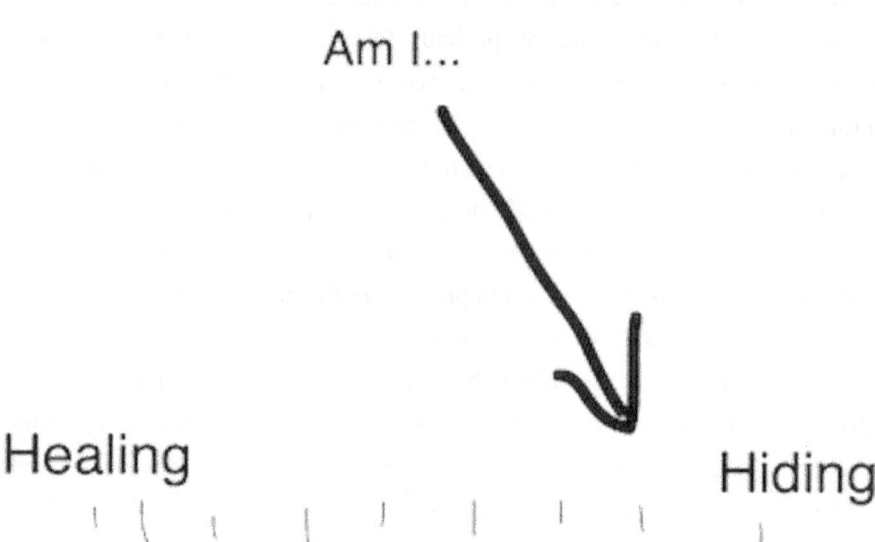

Figure 2.1 *The Isolation Gauge*

Perhaps this was bad timing? As I look back on it now, I am pretty sure it was bad timing.

For weeks before this, I had been trying to write. I wanted to work on another book. I wanted to figure out my website. I wanted to say, "I am still here!" *Perfect* was out. I had finished all my travels and signings. I had come home from the car wreck and collapsed in a heap, rested, and then rested some more. I might have been resting just a bit too much. I didn't write. I didn't talk much about the book tour. It felt like I had taken a painter's tarp and thrown it over my laptop, like my brain had some big project coming up, but all I could do was shroud the room in cloth, and maybe toss a few paintbrushes in the corner. I would look around, overwhelmed, shut the door, and tell myself, "I'll start tomorrow."

My ideas were thickly covered. And I had arrived at the retreat to uncover them. But that morning had been spent staring at my computer screen until I realized I needed a better light[2] for my room, and Target was just two blocks away. "I'll just get a lamp. That's all I need. And *then* I'll write."

An hour later, I had a shopping cart that was laden with half the snack aisle, two packs of La Croix Pamplemousse because it's the fancy one,[3] a lamp, two fuzzy guilt-blankets for my boys (they were on sale), and a whole lot of conflicted feelings. And then my phone pinged. It was a text from the school:

Hi! Happy Valley School District will be closing tomorrow and Friday to prepare, and on Monday, we will begin at-home learning. We are probably going to do this for the rest of your child's entire future. See your email for more information, and may God have mercy on us all. Make it a great day!

That text was paraphrased, by the way. I'm sure the original was way more professional, and I don't think there were any exclamation points because, you know, they didn't want to freak anybody out. But in my head, those exclamation points were there. And I wasn't. I wasn't *there*. I was in a Target, far away, trying to be all creative. In a pandemic.

If I had been in Walmart, they would have understood a breakdown. People do them there all the time. I looked at my cart with its stupid Oreo Thins and my stupid lamp and my stupid fizzy water, and I reached for my satchel. I was going to abandon my cart, head back to my room to pack, and go straight home.

And right then, I jumped because my phone rang. My friend Kate was calling me. We don't ever call each other—we text because children—but here she was *calling*. What's even weirder is that I answered. I never do that. Phone calls are weird. As I was already feeling weird, I decided to go with it and said, "Hello?"

She didn't even say hello back. She said this:

"You need to stay there." I looked around the aisle. "You need to stay there. Do not come home." My eyes filled up, and I stared up at Target's tall ceiling so I wouldn't drip all over the place. I think I spotted a little bird up there with a teeny tiny mask. Kate continued. "**Stay** there. It's ok, Dana. Brian is home. He's got this."

This was . . . possible? That's what my brain was telling me. Before I left, Brian had repeatedly told me, "Just go. You need this."[4] Brian is an engineer, which makes him strange to me. He is constantly finding what he calls "poor design" in our house and in our lives, and then commenting on it. Sometimes he fiddles with it. He views the world like it's full of glitches, nodding at them like, "I see you, glitch, and I'm just going to fix you." He's like a Spock who tells dad jokes. I see glitches in life and throw large tarps over them and just hope they'll go away.

For the past few weeks, Brian had been following the news like an engineer. Oh, there's an ominous situation looming on our horizon? It's poor design. We acknowledge. We maneuver. He had analyzed the situation, told me to stop obsessively reading about Covid-19 before bed, and then practically shoved me out the door to go to my retreat and write. "It'll be good for you," he said. "I'm here. The kids are all right." I didn't really believe him, but I also wanted to leave the house and the news and just go away.

I honestly didn't think we would really do the shelter-at-home thing. I just wanted to believe everything was just going to be ok. This is magical thinking, by the way, and I'm good at it.

Can I just tell you how fun it is to have married someone who is my complete opposite on the spectrum of dealing with life? Highly sensitive people marry Spock-y people all the time. It's like the universe is trying to make sure it stays balanced, I guess. Or God just likes a project. Either way, I am highly sensitive, and I quiver at a lot of things. But in this case, the overwhelm simply caused my brain to sort of blank out, and I froze, like an overwhelmed rabbit.

The brain will protect itself at all costs. If I'm being hit with too many stimuli, the part of my brain in charge of executive function just shuts down. If you're standing close to me when this happens, you can lean in and hear me go offline. Often, my overwhelm stems from a lack of control, which makes sense. Brian had more control. He was able to look at the facts (a school shutting down) and simply say, "I'm not going to get emotionally involved. What do we do next?"

I was barely able to read the text from the school before my emotions rushed in and blew things up.

That's why Kate called. She knew me so well that she guessed I would not be any good to my family in those first days. She didn't word it that way, as it is a slightly insulting thing to say to someone. She didn't offer this up:

"Hey. Stay there. You'll be a sh*t-show at home, anyhow." Besides, Kate has a master's degree in Christian Formation, and she would not have used a bad word. What she said instead was, "Hey. Stay there. Brian is fine, and you need to do this." Kate is a good friend.

I told her I'd think about it and then ended the call. People were still shopping. There was no rioting at Target. They were buying their lamps and their La Croix. Everyone looked kind of normal . . . except for the mask thing. Nobody else was crying. Maybe Kate was right.

I realize now that Kate was kind of right. And I also realize it's hard to admit that. It makes me a B mom instead of an A+ one. This is true. But one thing that Covid-19 taught me is that I will be a B mom sometimes,[5] and I will survive.

At home, Spock Dad would carry on. He would make the boys unhealthy lunches and tell them to go play basketball in the driveway instead of trying to check their mental state every five minutes.

I stayed. It was a Catholic retreat center, so it was very quiet, and there were a lot of pictures of Jesus around. One painting was of Mary holding what looked like a fifty-year-old baby Jesus with male-patterned balding. He greeted me every morning as I left my tiny room and headed to the large tables by the windows. "Hi balding Jesus," I would say to him, maybe not out loud, but I don't know. I hadn't talked to another soul for over three days. I did get some writing done, and I went on a lot of walks. I went home two days early, and I felt ready to tackle this new, scary thing. I also felt guilty as hell because what other mom had this luxury? Everybody was just dealing with a pandemic, and I had been walking around listening to water fountains and talking to balding Jesus. Kate had made me promise I would not feel guilty, so I tried. I did the best I could.

We all did the best we could.

When I got home on a Sunday, the boys would start official online school the next morning. And I dealt with this the best way I knew how. Lugging out a huge whiteboard that Brian had in his office, I created a color-coded schedule that managed our days within an inch of their lives. That whiteboard was a thing of beauty. It had lists of educational games for downtime. It posted all the schedules and teachers' emails. It had a bible verse on it. It was amazing. If we did what the whiteboard told us to, we would all be ok.

I do love a good list.

I was going to list *the crap out of* this situation.

My brain looked around the living room with its cute curtains and plants and the wide dining room table, and it said: "This is now going to be a place of learning, light, and peace. It will be school, but better!"

Yep, that's what my brain said. My executive function was all rested up, and now it was all: "Where's my clipboard? Go get whiteboard markers in a set of ten in assorted colors. Let's GOOOO"

So, here's a list for you:

Executive Function in the Brain

1. Self-monitors and keeps you aware
2. Manages emotions
3. Keeps you focused
4. Plans everything
5. Also, remembers stuff
6. Keeps you flexible, so you can bop around #1–5 with *ease*
7. Basically, it's that mom with the big purse who packs all the snacks and always has extra band-aids.

True story: I never had band-aids in my purse. Both my kids would ride bikes and play at parks, and I would be there, the mom, all willy-nilly with no band-aids, ever.

I did buy them; I just kept forgetting to put them in my purse. I am not a monster. I even had an emergency travel pack, but it stayed on the shelf in our bathroom closet because I kept forgetting to walk the fourteen steps with it to the car. There are so many skinned knees that went unattended because of this, but there was always another mom with proper first aid, and probably a fruit snack to administer if there was blood, and I just . . . let them. I didn't even feel all that guilty. I was not a band-aid mom. I was doing well if we remembered a water bottle, but even that was sketchy. When I was a kid, this constant lugging of water bottles everywhere was not a thing. When did this start? Why the constant need for hydration? I don't think I ever drank water as a kid. My mom had a constant pitcher of red Kool-Aid, and I drank that sometimes, then a glass of milk at dinner.

All this put me solidly in the B-category of caregiving. However, when we started at-home learning, I decided that *now* I was going to be a band-aid mom. I dragged the huge whiteboard thing into the dining room. I made a snack basket. I wiped down doorknobs and groceries and children. I was pivoting all over the place. The first couple of days I had my two boys journaling about their feelings, and we went on long walks together.

Then came week two.

One of the main causes of stress is an inability to control the environment around you. Stress is also caused by RNT and isolation.

In other words, Covid-19.

Here's another list:

Social Isolation and the Brain

1. Social isolation chips away at mental health.
2. This causes stress.
3. This leads to sleeping problems.
4. And then there's the heightened sense of fear.
5. This starts happening in weird places and times, like the park or a gas station. People film it.
6. There's also a bizarre increase in aggressiveness.
7. And all this just makes addictive habits try to help out because of what is happening.
8. It's *a lot*.

The slurry of Covid-19 and social isolation created something called the "double pandemic." It's a health crisis. The continued effects of being isolated from friends, family, medical aid, and more are not fully realized yet; researchers are just now breaching the surface of this phenomenon. But scientists have always known that isolation depletes physical and mental health. In one study, researchers found that prolonged isolation released a neurochemical that made mice get mad more quickly. The scientists saw the mice picking fights with other mice, then freezing in fear for much longer than necessary. Basically, these scientists were freaking out the mice, and the mice either got overly mad or overly scared. A mouse would get angry about its order at Starbucks and yell at the barista mouse about it, and then all the other mice would pull out their teeny tiny cell phones and start recording it while the first mouse shouted obscenities and stormed out. I just felt really bad for these angry mice and am hoping there was some scientist in there who eventually said, "Let's call this off and cuddle with them," but I've never gotten that vibe about scientists.

And, what if some of those mice also happened to be alcoholics?

Here's another list:

Alcoholism and the Pandemic

1. Binge drinking and addiction issues increased dramatically during the pandemic.
2. People in recovery have a higher risk of relapse due to the pandemic.
3. Unreported illnesses have increased post-pandemic.
4. Addiction is largely an unreported issue.
5. You do the math.

Here's some more math: Liquor stores in forty-seven out of fifty states remained open during the pandemic. They were deemed 94 percent essential.[6] Many states also relaxed additional rules around access to alcohol. West Virginia started allowing the sale of liquor in a to-go cup for all those call-up orders. My home state of Kansas passed a law in 2021 that made alcoholic to-go drinks a *permanent* thing. I am trying hard to withhold all major judgey statements because I'm sure I don't know all the rules here, but GO HOME, KANSAS. YOU ARE DRUNK. The plastic to-go containers are sealed with a sticker, though, so that makes it totally safe.

But liquor sales during the pandemic kept many restaurants from going under. Some small businesses needed the relaxed rules to survive. And so now we are here, in a post-Covid world where we stuck our toes in the water, so of course we want to be allowed to wander in deeper. We don't want that one lifeguard shrilling his whistle at us, telling us to get out of the water. We made this pool. Let us swim in it.

And it gets even more complicated. For those with severe alcohol dependencies, alcohol can be essential. Cold-turkey alcohol withdrawal can be deadly for those in pronounced stages of abuse, so cutting off sources could lead people who are suffering to do some really unsafe things. What about all those people who were in the throes of major alcohol use disorder during those early days of shutdown? What about all of them?

This all makes me think of my brother.

I write about my brother a lot. He has made an entrance in both of my previous books, and here he is again. I think Chris would tell me I'm beating the dead brother drum a bit too much, but he's dead, so he doesn't get a say.[7]

Chris was in and out of sobriety for the last ten years of his life. We all watched it. My parents tried to help. I did too. There he was, sometimes listening to the lifeguards, following the rules, but then . . . diving in again. And drowning.

The last time we had any real time with Chris was during his last attempt to stay sober. Mom and Dad moved him home, back to his downstairs bedroom, like he was a teenager again. He brought his clothes over in a plastic trash bag. And I can only wonder what it was like for him to lie in that bed in his old room and dry out. Did he stare at the ceiling and feel shame? A grown man, over fifty, trying to kick alcohol in his parents' basement? Or perhaps he felt relieved, or at least less afraid, to have this place to stay while he got through the first few days. The thing is, quitting cold turkey can be physically grueling because once you stop drinking heavily, your brain doesn't catch on right away. It had been so busy shoveling stimulants at us to keep up with all the depressants we had been guzzling that it was still in the zone, and nobody told it to cut it out.

When I got sober, nobody told my brain[8] for nearly two weeks about this huge thing I was doing for myself, which was tough.

My withdrawals were light in comparison to my brother's. There was vomiting and tremors, his heart was racing, and he was having chest pains and difficulty breathing. There might have been hallucinations or a fever, or seizures. He only talked to me about it one time, rather briefly, and after he explained some of it, he said, "Dana, I thought I was going to die." And that was it. I'm wondering now if he felt that chasm at the edge of his feet, venturing to explain something so painful to another person.

He did die from alcohol abuse about a year later, so I guess he was right.

Chris passed away from liver failure. He was in hospice, and when we arrived at his house during the last day of his life, I was horrified by what I saw. At the time, no one had been inside his home for over a year. He had completely cut us off by then. The floor by his bed was covered with stains. He had developed horrible eczema on his whole body; his bed was wretched. The kitchen, once his favorite place as a self-avowed foodie, was filthy. His house had become his drinking place, his fortress. A prison.

This is what alcohol can do. It took my handsome, hilarious brother, and it tore him up.

To clarify, Christopher and I are the same. I'm the same grade-A alcoholic that he was. I'm not any better than him, or any worse. I'm just the sober variety.

In April 2020, when the world shut down and our dining room became a school, I was in recovery, thank God. I had enough years of sobriety in me that drinking wasn't even on my mind. My southern friend Lisa would say, in her sweet drawl, "Drinking is no longer an option. Even if my ASS falls off." I was sober, and my ass and I were experiencing a whole new world together.

Oh, but also? I was ready to make the boys' pandemic as normal as possible.

I wanted to make sure they had *fun* during Covid, ok? I know. I don't know how else to say it. I had become a band-aid mom, and so we were going to be fine. It was fine. We were going to pull through. We were going to make blanket forts and go on nature walks and make some freakin' pandemic memories. Looking back on all that, I really wish I had been self-aware enough to realize how wackadoo all that sounds.

I was afraid, and I was trying to corner it.

Even after my short writing sabbatical with balding Jesus, I was again jonesing for control. I attached a lot of meaning to my colored markers and whiteboard, and it was around day three that I started monitoring my boys' moods like a psych ward nurse. My kids loved this. You can only ask your sons, "Hey, are you doing ok? How are you *feeling*? Do you miss your friends? Do you want a hug?" a few times before they get monosyllabic.

I did bake a whole lot of cookies. I felt so helpless, and so I baked at it.

Nothing says love like ordering five bags of chocolate chips from Walmart and then silently crying while you wipe the bags down with Clorox wipes, until one son comes into the kitchen, eyes this, and backs slowly out of the room.

I hunkered down and sheltered in place, and I joked about how introverts were secretly loving this. I didn't feel lonely. I had two boys and four pets smooshed up against me every day. There wasn't physical room for loneliness.

This is true. I wasn't lonely. I was isolated.

Isolation dries out the brain. If I socially invest in others, my neural pathways perk up and bloom. Cognitive skills like building empathy, practicing self-control, mental processing, and planning are all strengthened by social bonding. Take that all away, and those neural circuits wither.

Simply put: more bonding = more braining.

Social isolation also depletes endorphins. It sucks the joy out of you. Chimps know this. They practice grooming behaviors for the specific purpose of physically touching the gross furriness of their companion. This closeness releases endorphins, which allows the chimpanzees to build cognitive function and self-preservation. Also, there's a snack.

Maybe I was doing better with the endorphins by baking all those cookies, but I wasn't bonding with my boys. I wanted to. But after that first week, most of our time sheltering in place shifted to survival. The lists slowly got covered up or frayed. The plans for fresh air and industry devolved into screens and naps. There were a lot of carbs.

Surviving is not fun. It was not built for fun. Survival is about getting through it alive.

A final list:[9]

Alcohol Use During Covid-19

1. Alcohol consumption has increased in nearly every state since the pandemic.
2. People on average now consume 2.8 gallons of alcohol per year; that's almost 600 drinks and a 6.6 percent increase.
3. Alcohol-related deaths have increased in every state, and some states are seeing deaths nearly double.

In the spring of 2021, the mask mandate ended. People were slowly crawling out of their homes. It was a little weird to go to the store and wear lip gloss again. I felt like the entire lower portion of my face was pale and soft, but that could also be because of all those cookies.

At some point in May, I took my car into the shop because it was making a weird noise. This noise had been going on for quite a few weeks, but I was unused to going places and talking to people about things, so I played my favorite game: Putting It Off Because Maybe It Will Just Go Away. One evening, I made the mistake of mentioning the weird noise to my husband, Brian the Engineer. What followed was such a dizzying barrage of engineer-y questions that I answered "I don't know . . . maybe?" fourteen times until it was suggested I get the car in to see Kevin, our mechanic. We were also long overdue for an oil change, so I was brave and set up the appointment.

Kevin is one of those people you can talk to about your life, or your car's weird noises, or any combination of both. He is ready to talk cars, but also about your hopes and dreams, you know? I had forgotten this. So when I showed up that day, he made me feel right at home, or as right at home as one could feel in the waiting room that has bad coffee in styrofoam cups and a lot of magazines about hunting.

I handed over the keys, and then I sort of muttered, "Um, also? Could you check out this weird noise that my car is making?" For some reason, I didn't want to offend Kevin by asking him a car question. Maybe he wasn't feeling like a mechanic that day. I don't know. I don't like springing things on people.

Kevin leaned in and asked what I dreaded: "Sure. What kind of noise?"

It all came down to this. This was the moment. At some point, I knew I would have to perform the noise, and my trial run with Brian had been a disaster.

"A sort of whirring? And then a scerreeeerrch at the end of the whir. Like, there's a bird in there?"

I didn't really add the bird part because it seemed silly. But the car did sound like an asthmatic bird had decided to ride along with me until I had to talk to Kevin about it. I felt sheepish and mumbled something about being hesitant to mention it. But then I added, "I was just getting kind of scared to drive my car, actually. What if something is really wrong?"

Kevin nodded. "It's probably the double transductor. Probably lost its vortex thermometer because the catastrophic comptroller is off." I am making this part up because I don't remember what was wrong with the car. I only remember that he fixed the noise, and I drove it home that day.

What I DO remember is that he said this:

"You should always ask. Driving is day-to-day stuff. And nobody should have to do day-to-day stuff, scared."

When Covid sent us home, and when we watched the news and heard about the numbers, or experienced the death and pain of it firsthand, we were also trying to do the day-to-day stuff. We were making meals, doing school and working, and paying bills. For me? I was doing it scared. I was doing it terrified. Even making a meal would cause me to pause and wonder about the germs. I forgot to wipe the groceries; had I now introduced this awful thing into their *food*? After I had bleached the kitchen and myself, I would worry that I hadn't made the meal healthy enough. And the boys weren't getting enough exercise. Oh, and their brains would be mush because of all the screens. There were many screens going on.

I wondered if life was always going to be like this. I was full to the brim with simmering fear. For at least a full year, I was afraid. It takes a toll.

Kevin's solution was simple. Reach out. Ask for help. But I never did. I never told anyone how scared I was—probably because I wasn't really acknowledging it myself. I didn't talk about it because I looked around and saw people wearing masks and doing their day-to-day, and they seemed ok. There was no crying in the bread aisle.

I cried in the bread aisle once. No one noticed because most of the snot was contained behind the mask, which was gross but helpful.

I know that this sounds ridiculous. I know other people were just as scared as I was. But I was isolated. Isolation messes with your mind. I had all these *feelings* about what was going on, like I was carrying them around in my hands, waiting for someone to help offload them, like Julia Roberts with all her wads of cash in *Pretty Woman*.

And I know that this compares me to a prostitute (with a heart of gold), so the analogy is a bit wobbly. But I just keep seeing that snobby sales clerk in the movie, eyeing me as I shyly approach, holding out my excess emotions and needing help. She gives me the up and down and then turns me away. Isolation turned me away.

Besides, our family was healthy, and we were managing. We were ok. I should be grateful. I should be. We were safe at home.

I kept quiet.

Big mistake. *Huge.*

Notes

1. Correction. He did not want to marry **me**. He went right smack into another relationship after we broke up and married her. Not that we should have ever gotten married at all. Like ever. But I at least wanted a decent amount of lag time before he hitched up to a girl that looked just like me. Did I stalk him on the internet to find all this out? Of course I did. Incidentally, he also named his first son Henry, which is my youngest son's name and I SEE WHAT YOU'RE DOING RYAN YOU NEED TO GET OVER ME. Also, Brian if you are reading this right now, you are the straight up best husband ever. We can talk later about this footnote but you are so hot.

2. I am married to a man who turns on overhead lights when he enters a room. I then tut at him and flit around the perimeter, clicking on the seven small lamps we have all ready to go to make sure the room is cozy. I once told him overhead lighting made me think of gynecological exams, and he blinked at me a lot. It's fine. He wasn't able to make the leap between a light fixture and women's health, and that's all right. But I will continue to festoon my house with forty-seven small and tasteful lamps because nobody needs a gyno in their living room.

3. Calm down, La Croix, it's just grapefruit. You called all your other flavors by their names. Orange was just orange. Black current was, you guessed it, black currant. But grapefruit? I don't know what happened with you. Perhaps you had just finished your

Duolingo practice for the day, and you got all cocky about it, and told all the folks at the marketing meeting: "Forget grapefruit, guys . . . Let's go: PAMPLEMOUSSE!!" and all the marketers nodded because they didn't want to look uncultured.

4   It is not lost on me that people were basically pushing me out of my house here. I asked Brian if he ever looked forward to time away from me when I would go on speaking gigs, and he answered, "No. I need you by my side at all times," without looking up from the game, and I love him for that.

5   Often.

6   Libraries were not.

7   I firmly believe that Chris has no problem with me writing about him. I really do. He would not wish this disease on anyone, and also? Writing about him makes me feel close to him. I miss my brother.

8   I had about a solid week of feeling extremely nauseous and achy, like I had the flu. My thoughts were loud and kept crashing about, and they didn't make much sense. It's like I had my own rage metal withdrawal band in my head screaming at me during random moments of my day. The band sounded like this: "THIS! WON'T! WORK! BECAUSE! YOU! SUCK." I slept a lot to avoid the band. It would have been really nice if instead my brain would have been all congratulatory and proud of me, like "Girrll! You are ahmazzzing!" but my brain has never talked to me like that in my entire life.

9   Alternative title for this chapter: I Like Big Lists and I Cannot Lie.

Bibliography

1   **By the end of 2022, forty percent of us rated our stress levels as "fair to poor":** American Psychiatric Association. (2022, December 21). Americans Anticipate Higher Stress at the Start of 2023 and Grade Their Mental Health Worse. https://www.psychiatry.org/news-room/news-releases/americans-anticipate-higher-stress-at-the-start-of#:~:text=More%20than%20one%20in%20four,percentage%20points%20from%20last%20yea.

2   **If I'm being hit with too many stimuli, the part of my brain in charge of executive function just shuts down:** Bekkali, S. (2023, April 25). What Is the Science Behind "Overwhelm"?. *modo.* https://www.meetmodo.com/post/what-is-the-science-behind-overwhelm#:~:text=What%20is%20the%20science%20behind%20this%20feeling%3F,function%E2%80%9D%20(EF)%20capacities.

3   **Social isolation and the brain:** California Institute of Technology. (2018, May 17). How Social Isolation Transforms the Brain. *ScienceDaily*. Retrieved October 8, 2023 from www.sciencedaily.com/releases/2018/05/180517113856.htm.

4 **The slurry of Covid-19 and social isolation created something called the "double pandemic":**
California Institute of Technology. (2018, May 17). How Social Isolation Transforms the Brain. *ScienceDaily*. Retrieved October 8, 2023 from www.sciencedaily.com/releases/2018/05/180517113856.htm.

5 **... researchers found that prolonged isolation released a neurochemical that made mice get mad more quickly.**
Dajose, L. (2018, May 17). *How Social Isolation Transforms the Brain*. California Institute of Technology. https://www.caltech.edu/about/news/how-social-isolation-transforms-brain-82290.

6 **Binge drinking and addiction issues increased dramatically during the pandemic:**
Chacon, N. C., N. Walia, A. Allen, A. Sciancalepore, J. Tiong, R. Quick, S. Mada, M. A. Diaz, and I. Rodriguez (2021). Substance Use During Covid-19 Pandemic: Impact on the Underserved Communities. *Discoveries (Craiova, Romania)* 9 (4): e141. https://doi.org/10.15190/d.2021.20.

7 **People in recovery have a higher risk for relapse due to the pandemic:**
Yazdi, K., I. Fuchs-Leitner, J. Rosenleitner, and N. W. Gerstgrasser (2020, November 24). Impact of the Covid-19 Pandemic on Patients with Alcohol Use Disorder and Associated Risk Factors for Relapse. *Frontiers*. https://www.frontiersin.org/articles/10.3389/fpsyt.2020.620612/full.

8 **Unreported illnesses have increased post-pandemic:**
Ducharme, J. (2023, February 27). Patient Burnout is a Simmering Public Health Crisis. *Time*. https://time.com/6257775/patient-burnout-health-care/

9 **Addiction is largely an unreported issue:**
Boniface, S., J. Kneale, and N. Shelton (2014). Drinking Pattern Is More Strongly Associated with Under-Reporting of Alcohol Consumption than Socio-Demographic Factors: Evidence from a Mixed-Methods Study. *BMC Public Health* 14: 1297. https://doi.org/10.1186/1471-2458-14-1297.

10 **Liquor stores in 47 out of 50 states remained open during the pandemic:**
Gerndt, E. (2021, May 19). Is Alcohol Essential? Lessons from Covid-19 on How Policy Impacts Access. *Counter Tools*. https://countertools.org/blog/is-alcohol-essential-lessons-from-covid-19-on-how-policy-impacts-access/.

11 **GO HOME KANSAS YOU ARE DRUNK:**
Chung, R. (2021, May 21). What to Know About Kansas' New Liquor Law: To-Go Cocktails, Beer & More. *KSNT 27 News*. https://www.ksnt.com/capitol-bureau/what-to-know-about-kansas-new-liquor-law-to-go-cocktails-beer-more/#:~:text=Under%20the%20new%20law%2C%20restaurants,half%20a%20gallon%20in%20beer.

12 **For those with severe alcohol dependencies, alcohol can be essential:**
Tiako, M. J. N., and K. C. Priest (2020, April 7). Yes, Liquor Stores are Essential Businesses. *Scientific American Blog Network*. https://tinyurl.com/y6yjjxe4.

13 **... once you stop drinking heavily, your brain doesn't catch on right away:**
Amelia, S. (2023, August 16). Alcohol Withdrawal Symptoms, Timeline & Detox Treatment. *American Addiction Centers*. https://americanaddictioncenters.org/withdrawal-timelines-treatments/alcohol.

14 I wasn't lonely. I was isolated:
Bzdok, D., and R. I. M. Dunbar (2022). Social Isolation and the Brain in the Pandemic Era. *Nature Human Behaviour* 6: 1333–43. https://doi.org/10.1038/s41562-022-01453-0.

15 Alcohol Use During Covid-19:
Gilbert, C., D. Ovalle, and H. Zakharenko (2023, July 17). Alcohol Consumption Surged During the Pandemic—and Deaths Followed. *The Washington Post*. https://www.washingtonpost.com/wellness/2023/07/13/alcohol-consumption-deaths.

3

I'm Hungry

After fifty years of hating my body, I am tired.

It all began in junior high gym class. And really, what doesn't?

Our school required that we wear stretchy one-piece gym suits because it was the 1980s, and junior high wasn't traumatic enough on its own. The suits were a dark navy with a wide white elastic band around the waist and neck. In the summer before seventh grade, my mom took me to the uniform place to buy one, and I pulled it on in the changing booth and then stared silently at the mirror under the fluorescent lighting. "Let's take a look," my mom called, and I opened the door and stood in front of more mirrors. Mom clucked and pulled at the fabric around my thighs and then asked me to turn around.

"Mom, it's huge," I said. To which she tugged at the sleeve and answered,

"That's good. We want there to be room to grow."

What happened was, I grew. In late summer before eighth grade, I knew Mom wouldn't buy me a new grade gym suit. "Why would we get a new one, honey?" she asked. "You have a perfectly good suit that fits you just fine." I nodded, thinking that it probably would fit just fine. Probably. Good money was spent on that suit, and for all I knew it was perfectly fine.

On the first day of gym class in eighth grade, I found the opposite was true. My gym locker was next to Kristy Harper's and about four of her entourage. Kristy was tall, tan, and popular, with a side ponytail and a mean streak. I tended to stay quiet and just listen to Kristy; she talked incessantly, usually about boys, and I found her fascinating and terrifying. Being around her always made me feel like I didn't quite know where to stand or how to make my face look.

I pulled on the gym suit. It was snug. And that's when I heard the snicker. The girls were staring, and as I stood up, I noticed that Kristy's gym suit draped around her, slung low on her hips, loose and slouchy. And she said, "Is that *last* year's suit?" like my gym suit was a fashion faux pas. This is redundant. It was a *gym suit*.

Kristy's suit, however, looked, dare I say it? Stylish. As she carefully removed her add-a-bead necklace and placed it in her locker, her collarbones jutted. She had gathered the waist of the blue fabric with a day-glow green scrunchie. She wore Tretorns and had no problems.

How do I go home and say all this to my mom? How do I try to explain the green scrunchie? My mom was just as uncool as I am. We had solidarity that way. How do I tell her that how this blue thing fits me was directly proportional to my survival of eighth grade? I had no idea that the 1983 Fall gym suit's style would be billowy. Who keeps up with this stuff?

The blue suit nestled up in my crotch for 186 days that year, while I tried to climb a rope to the ceiling with only a two-inch-thick mat to catch me if I fell. I made it three feet up the rope before I started to slowly sliiide back down, and the suit crawled up into places where it had no business.

At the end of class, we would all hustle back into the locker room, and I would silently peel it off and throw it in my locker. Kristy had a pink bra. I think it was leopard print. Mine was white, one-ply, and had a tiny pink rosette in the middle. I really hated gym class.

After school, I would get home, sigh heavily, and burrow into the fridge for a snack. Then I would head downstairs. For a long time, I was really into applesauce and Nilla wafers. Then I started a cold nacho cheese and chips thing. Then, buttered saltines. My snacks had a few courses and were accompanied by large tumblers of red Kool-Aid. This was part of the routine. The basement of our house was cool and quiet. It has dark wood paneling and a maroon leather chair that was known as That's Dad's Spot Don't Sit There. He wasn't home, so I would plunk down, the leather squeaking lovingly around me, throw my legs across the side, and watch *Gilligan's Island*. And I would eat. I found out later that this was called decompression. Back then, I called it necessary.

Middle school was when I realized I was not cool. This wasn't that important to me. I knew I would never be popular. I didn't have the clothing budget for that. What was crucial, however, was that people liked me. Being uncool was ok, as long as people thought I was nice about it. But for some reason, being uncool now also meant you were awful, and I didn't get it. So, I made it my mission to be the nicest person to everyone, all the time. I would continue on this niceness plan for the next thirty years of my life. It was exhausting, but I was really nice about it.

In ninth-grade Honors English class, I also realized that my head was too big. This was because I sat behind Laura Sinclair. Laura had long, silky hair that she wore in a swishy ponytail, and it swished my papers off my desk daily. That ponytail had a life of its own. Laura's head was small and delicate. I should know because I stared at it for a full hour every day of my ninth-grade year. My head, in comparison, was this lumbering thing. My ponytail did not swish. It stuck out from my gigantic skull. Laura's beauty was directly proportional to the swish of her ponytail. Occasionally, she would actually take out the ponytail with one silky tug on her scrunchie, and every boy in the room would cross his legs. I watched as she would lean back, almost into my lap it seemed, and gather it up again. Her hair would slip through her hand in one solid ribbon; I could almost hear the soft hiss of it as it pooled, liquid and well-behaved, into her hands. There were so many good genes involved in this whole ritual that *Seventeen Magazine* started calling her mother right then. And for 186 days, I sat there behind her and wondered how I could lose weight from my head.

I never found out what happened to Laura. I didn't keep in touch with many of my high school colleagues, but imagine her, perched on a chair, saying things like, "Um, it's a bit warm here? I'm glistening," which is something Laura actually told our teacher, Mr. Boley, back in our stuffy classroom. That kind of stuff stays with you. Air-conditioned schools were not a thing in the 1980s, but hard-as-nails popularity was.

I'm wondering if Laura is a Tiny Mom today. You know who they are. They have the bone structure of Bella Hadid, but they also have four kids. Each child's name starts with an H, and they are all strikingly beautiful and a little bit mean. Tiny Moms have big key chains and talk about pilates. Their cheekbones are sharp. Little birds could come down and alight on those cheekbones, which would look weird, but a Tiny Mom would make it work. "Oh, these old things?" she would smile if someone asked about the birds, "I've had these forever!" Their jean size is in the single digits, and lo, it has always been so. When Tiny Moms stand up, they don't take a minute to pull up or adjust or suck in. They just walk around in the air, without any consequences. And, most mysterious of all, they can wear sleeveless shirts even in their fifties. Tiny Moms are all related to Laura Sinclair.

There is no way I would ever be able to be a Tiny Mom. Even if I weighed the same, I would still not weigh the same.

In college, I guzzled Slim Fast and took my roommate's diet pills. I ate cereal three times a day with watery skim milk. I also started drinking.

In my twenties, I discovered baby carrots. They helped me handle low-rise jeans. If my waistline seemed a bit poochy, I would make homemade melba toast and snack on it, sometimes with a thin smear of sugar-free jam as a treat to curb cravings. By the way, homemade melba toast is bread that you bake at a low temperature in the oven for hours until it becomes like lava rock, and then, as you eat it, it's so noisy that you have to slow down or you will get a headache.

In the 1990s, Jen and I did Weight Watchers and learned to count everything as a point. Apples? two points. An egg? one point. Low-fat skim milk string cheese? one point. I ate a lot of string cheese. One time I was out to eat with friends, and I was hungry.[1] The waiter brought a chaotic platter of nachos, laden with glistening cheese and chips and guacamole, and I wilted in despair. How was I going to tabulate all this? The mental math involved made eating feel like a fourth-grade times-table speed test. *Figure this **out**, I thought as I stared at the pile of chips and cheese, my friends all reaching for all the extra-gooey bits. *I'm starving.*

I was constantly thinking about food. Did you know? Coffee creamer is one point if you measure it into a tablespoon instead of just glugging it into the mug. And a stick of gum, as long as it's sugar-free, has ZERO points. I would go through entire packs of gum in an afternoon. Bless. Also, don't eat bananas because they're a whopping three points, so they're unhealthy.

In my thirties, I feared pregnancy because it would make me pack on pounds, aka *a baby*, and I ran three miles a day up to my eighth month because of this. On my final run, I tripped and fell, and we had to go to the hospital to check on the baby. (Charlie is now sixteen and very ok, but as soon as he reads this, he's going to use it against me. I love you, son.) When we were done with the examination, the nurse handed me paper towels to wipe off the gel stuff, and she looked at my face and said, "How about we try walking?" We did.

In my forties, I bought diet books that told you they weren't diet books. "It's not a diet; it's a way of life!" the books said. I lived so many lives back then. These diets had you mix certain types of food with other types of food and buy lots of almond flour and xanthan gum. Did you know you can add okra to brownies, which makes them taste kind of . . . green? And then you eat half the pan because they don't really satisfy, but still, it's dessert?

In my forties, I also got sober. And because of that, I turned a page to a very new and exciting chapter of my life called "I Don't Have Time for Any More Bullshit." This translated into my issues with food, in a good way, for the first time. Early sobriety, as we all know, clangs a loud craving bell, and so I ate the sugar. I had a thing for grape Blow Pops and kept a large bag of them by my bedside, in the kitchen, and about five were always shoved in the console of my car. And it was ok. Early sobriety trumps sugar. Sobriety is the most important thing.

And then, for a long time, sobriety got a lot easier. But after a while, sugar started to get harder. It's complicated.

Here is an example: It's been a stressful day. I'd started having issues with sleeping. My husband leaves for a work trip, so at around 5 p.m. I decided to call him to check that he didn't die in a fiery plane crash. If he's on a work trip and I have not heard from him in a few hours, my brain does this: "It must be a fiery plane crash. That's why he hasn't called. The boys and I are going to end up in a van down by the river." Also, even if he hasn't died in a fiery plane crash, I know that Brian doesn't love me as much as I love him because he hasn't called first. So, either way, I'm screwed. I finally trudge through all my neuroses and give him a call, and he picks up after two rings. I am not a widow. But now I'm resentful. It's confusing.

Brian says, "Hey, babe! How's my sweetie?" His words are buoyant, and I narrow my eyes. From across the miles, I can hear it. Brian has a beer voice. Now I'm more resentful. First of all, I was almost a widow. Second, I love him more than he loves me. And now, he has the audacity to drink when I cannot.

Food. Food was my second thought after the plane crash. "Well," my brain says, slapping my knees, "Who's hungry?" And right there, that's when the thinking stops. Anxiety and addiction are dysfunctional siblings. Anxiety stands at the starting line of my mind, waiting for a feeling to fire the starting gun. That night, it was this conversation with my husband that pulled the trigger. My friend, Mindy, who is thirty-seven years sober, always tells me, "First thought wrong." I do have to congratulate myself that after hearing Brian's beer voice, my first thought was not, "Let's drink at this. You are uncomfortable and stressed. Bring on thirteen glasses of wine." That thought did not happen.

Instead, my first thought was "Well, let's go for food. Nobody else has issues with food after they get sober, right?"

My binge starts in my brain. It has nothing to do with my stomach. There is no hunger, only feelings. The brain starts to feel stress and shifts in its seat, muttering, "Uh, I'm getting uncomfortable. Could we have some dopamine over here? I don't do stress." Ben and Jerry, camped out in the freezer, laconically raise their hands and say, "Dude. We're here for you." And my brain, always willing to go for the quickest option because it hates waiting, says, "Ah yes! That has always worked in the past! I have been grooving to this for ages. It is super effective." Somewhere, buried deep in my prefrontal cortex, a bit of tired mumbling says, "Um, actually not so much really," but after the first hit of sugar, my brain turns off. Like an old TV, it just clicks and the screen shudders to a pinprick of light, then black. Sugar pulls the plug. When the Snickers bar or the ice cream or the bagel hits my system, I don't even get a groan of pleasure. There's . . . nothing. This, incidentally, is an enormous relief.

And this is why a binge is so very difficult to ward off. I would like to think my brain is super attentive to me and all my needs, but in this case, my brain zones out like when I drive for twenty minutes and then realize I have no recollection of how I got to my destination.

Oh, and willpower? It's useless (Figure 3.1).

I'm Hungry

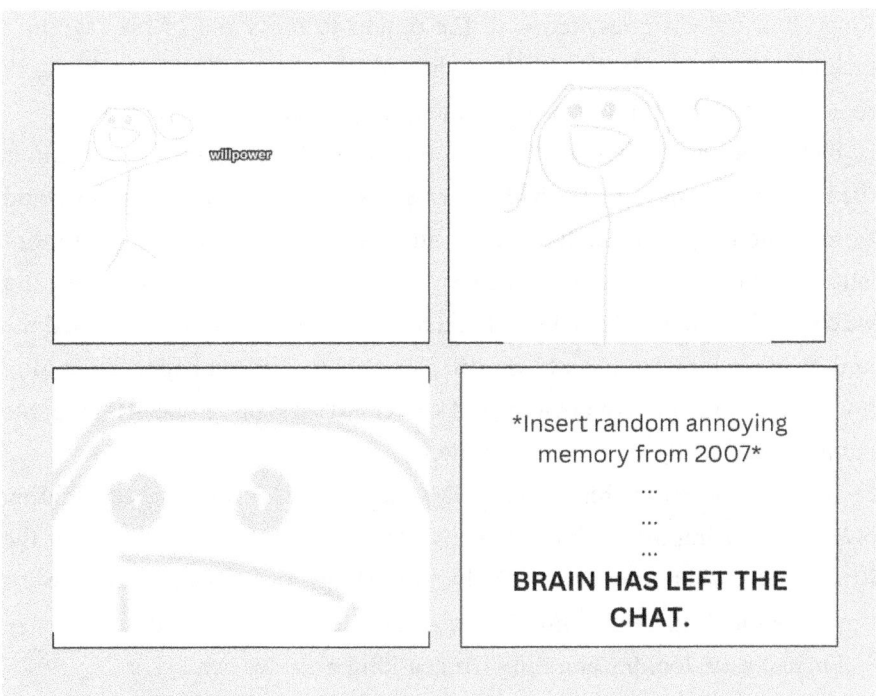

Figure 3.1 *Willpower Never Works*

Sugar. It fires up my brain very much like a glass of wine does. The alcohol took all feelings of inadequacy, shame, and dread, and switched them off. Sugar does the same. My brain likes a repetitive groove.

Let's say you take a rat, name him Ralph, and feed him a lot of sugar. This rat lives in a small square cage with fluorescent lighting. Ralph's dwelling has no ambiance. It's pretty unpleasant, even if you are a rat. The most fun for Ralph is his wheel. If Ralph wants to work out, he can whirl himself around on it a couple of times, which is a bit of a thrill, but it's short-lived. If he's super bored, he can chew up a toilet paper roll. Ralph also only gets crunchy brown pebbles for lunch and dinner. Since Ralph is vastly more intelligent than anyone ever gives him credit for, Ralph knows his circumstances are less than ideal. So, when presented with a Ring Ding, Ralph takes a bite and immediately stops caring about the harsh lighting, his lack of a nice couch or cozy throw pillows, or that the water in his dispenser is never chilled. He is hit with a dopamine surge that makes his little paws scrabble for more Ring Ding. He wants only

Ring Ding now. If presented with the option to move out of his cage to a nice three-bedroom with a fireplace, he only wants the Ring Ding. He can't remember what it feels like **not** to want a Ring Ding.

By the way, we did this exact experiment when I was in third grade, minus the three-bedroom cage. We had two rats, and all the kids brought junk food from home to give to the lucky rat. Our teacher fed the healthy rat a lot of lettuce. We treated our soon-to-be very obese rat to Cookie Crisp cereal, and we cheered when one day, a kid offered his lunchtime Twinkie. We named the junk food rat Templeton, and I am still haunted by whatever happened to him. It was 1977, and I guess eight-year-old kids could mess up rats back then in the name of science. It was a different time.

So, am I the rat in this scenario? My cage has a lot more accent lighting because that's important, but other than that, I think I'm the rat. I want the Ring Dings. When presented with the Ring Dings, I will forget about the last time I ate the Ring Dings, and I felt so gross and shaky afterward.

I'm just a rat, looking at a Ring Ding, asking it to love her.

I had a routine with drinking, and I had a routine with food. Both begin and end the same. My addictions are the most consistent things in my life. There is the trigger; in this case, the husband who is buzzed. Because of the husband with a beer voice, my brain starts slowly circling me. I walk from room to room, putting away things, moving a book, or patting the dog. Most triggers don't occur at work or out of the house—my house seems to be a fortress for Ok, Let's Do This. It's a place of control, where my environment is curated to allow for failure. In public, I put triggers away into a small hamster corral that I shut the lid on and dim the lights, and my brain tells them, "Sleep, little hamsters. I'll let you out as soon as I get home and into something with an elastic waistband."

I walk into the kitchen. The hamsters scrabble about in my head, and because they are sociable, they all start to talk to each other and to me.

Friends, I know we have talked about rodents a lot in this chapter, but I have never trusted a hamster in my life. One hamster says, "She's in the kitchen. She's eyeing the chips. It's not looking good." And another one answers, "She is not going to do a binge. Absolutely not. Carrots and hummus. Do they still make SlimFast? Nothing yummy. Like, ever." Meanwhile, one other hamster whisks out a small bistro table and unfurls a checked tablecloth. He plunks down a drippy candle in a Chianti bottle and says, "For this evening's special, there is fourteen-month-old garlic bread in the freezer."

I listen to all the hamsters. I really do. But, I start with the garlic bread.

For me, a binge must be done with the couch and a movie. It's Netflix and fill.[2] There must be lots of cozy blankets and no observers, very little cutlery or table manners. Usually, a dog is smooshed on my feet. This could mask itself as self-care. There's nothing wrong with a blanket and a dog, and Ben and Jerry's. I need to relax! It's comfort food! There's a dog here!

I tidy a corner of a table. I grab a blanket. I find the remote. I pat the dog. Hosmer sighs, and as I bring in the garlic bread and sit down, he jumps and curls his little body tightly against me. *Look, I don't endorse this*, he says. *But I'll stay close because there are crumbs. Also, I love you, but you are making really poor decisions.*

Garlic bread in the air fryer is the gateway drug. Then I need something sweet to combat the carbs, so I go hunting for Ben & Jerry's, always a great choice. Ice cream smooths the way for something crunchy, so I dig in the pantry for those healthy sesame crackers that taste like sticks. Next, it's time for something sour and chewy. I find stale Starbursts from my sons' Easter candy stash.

Then, there is a feeling of "Well what the hell you've screwed it all up now. Let's just eat a full sleeve of saltines until you're surrounded by white shards." The dog shoots me a pitying glance and silently snuffs up the crumbs. At some point, I find that the only brain activity I have left is deciding what food shall journey with me from the kitchen back to the couch. I take things one at a time, and each item is a little less prepared, a little less inviting. I end up with a stale popsicle from the depths of the freezer.

If I keep eating, I don't have to think. And finally, bed beckons. I'm so tired. I'm shaky from all the sugar. And of course, sleep is not going to happen because my hormones and pretty much any other physiological process in my body have been hijacked. I try to get comfortable with a bunch of pillows to prop me up, and I scroll on my phone until 1 a.m. The next morning, my body aches; my joints scream as I head downstairs. I am a failure. I am pathetic and small. I am huge and ashamed. I circle myself as both the least and the most important person in my world.

I vow: Never again.

Because I am so strung out and tired from last night's binge, I feel rotten all day. Because I feel rotten, I don't move my body. Because I don't move my body, I don't crave a salad. One hamster, let's call him Jesse, says, "And I'm really feeling like a Snickers right now. You can start a diet on Monday." And the process starts all over again. Sugar shuts down feelings, and within about thirty minutes, it also starts to shut down all the alert chemicals in my brain, and I become terribly, ridiculously, horribly tired.

This mirrors depression, which scares me, and my anxiety kicks in. Before you know it, all those addiction grooves are activated, and my brain is in dread mode. The hamsters shrug and scuttle off; this has happened before, and it will happen again. It's nearly time for their nap.

It's . . . it's just like the drinking. It's just like it was for me back in 2014. There are no empty plastic bottles of vodka stashed in my closet, but the same feelings are stockpiled up there. And there is one tiny hamster, Walter, who remains. He's a quiet one who sits in the back. He points his tiny paw at me. "This is just like 2014. It's 2014 but with crinkly wrappers." He sighs deeply and steeples his little paws. Then he leans forward, *What if all these feelings mean you are going to drink again, Dana?*

I could stop it right there, but I don't. I get up, find a stale bag of Tostitos, and finish my second binge in two days with tortilla crumbs and salsa. The chips are loud, and they drown out Walter. The crumbs mock me as I wipe them away from my shirt and the couch. Who knew that a tortilla chip could carry the weight of my sobriety? Who knew I could give a corn chip that much power?

When I was a kid, I remember my parents as behind-the-door fighters. My dad had been sober since I was little. I don't know if this had any input on the style of argument in the house, but I remember that when I heard them walk down the hall and shut that bedroom door, a pall of gloom would descend. My sister and I would tiptoe around and say things like, "Is Dad mad? How long have they been in there? Did we do something?" And it seemed like hours that they would remain in the bedroom. Occasionally, we would hear a muffled, raised voice, and my entire body would tense up. I would freeze, willing myself and the whole house to just be quiet, to be peaceful. It felt like they would stay behind that heavy door for the rest of my childhood. Or, that only one parent would emerge, the other lost forever into the unknown.

And somehow, there would be this conviction that if I were really quiet and really good, that door might open sooner. My silent goodness carried that much responsibility. I felt like the bedroom door stood about ten feet tall. I would slowly tiptoe past it, silently willing it to open, but also dreading it doing so. And sometimes I would sneak down the dark carpeted hall and descend the stairs to our basement. My dad was a sales broker for Hostess Bakeries, and stashed away in our freezer was about a year's supply of Zingers. I would find them and then go hide in our back storage place under the stairs, by the play kitchen and a cat box, and I would tear open the packages. They smelled of vanilla and freezer burn, and I gnawed through the brittle frosting and the frozen cake and all the feelings. It was dark and quiet, and I felt safe.

By the way, my parents are still very happily married. This October will be their sixtieth wedding anniversary. Their marriage is stitched together with exasperation, patience, and deep love; it has a patina to it, of two people who have been able to spend the majority of their lives with their best friend.

The last time I visited Mom and Dad, I was helping them with dinner, and my mom asked me to go down to the freezer and fetch something. As I opened the heavy lid and stared inside, I felt myself peering around. There were no Zingers. They had been replaced by forty foil-wrapped tiny packages of random leftovers, some as small as the palm of my hand. There were tiny little labeled squares of "oyster dressing" or "Eckrich ssg" or, disconcertingly, "mush."[3] Nothing remotely sweet and Hostess-like, not even hidden below tiny packages of sliced cheese and a quarter bag of Triscuits. The freezer had become a smorgasbord of tiny eats for tiny old people. I guess my parents had learned that Hostess Zingers pale in comparison to "chik alf." Everybody knows that.

"Where's the Zingers?" I jokingly asked as I ascended the stairs. Mom looked confused for a moment, then laughed. "We haven't had a Zinger down there since you two were kids."

So, after the phone call with Brian and his beer voice, when all the feelings show up and I am adrift, I think that little girl shows up too. My prefrontal cortex does try to lecture me about this. It tries. But, really, who wants to make that little girl feel bad? Eventually, my prefrontal cortex throws up its gray hands and gives up. The grooves are too deep. The hallway is too long. The door slams shut. Food issues? C'mon. It's no big deal. It's not vodka, for Pete's sake. It's not important enough. Or problematic enough. It's not loud enough. It's just *Zingers*.

And as I shake out the remaining crumbs of tortilla chips into my hand and stare at them, my stomach hurts. I find myself getting up, looking, actually looking to see if there is something else, anything really, that I can eat so I won't be able to ask if this is finally enough.

And I realize. This is killing me. Just enough.

Notes

1 I was always hungry.

2 I'm sorry.

3 Mushrooms sauteed in butter and garlic. Everyone should have this in their freezer.

Bibliography

1 **Anxiety and addiction are dysfunctional siblings:**
Cox, B. J., G. R. Norton, R. P. Swinson, and N. S. Endler (1990). Substance Abuse and Panic-Related Anxiety: A Critical Review. *Behaviour Research and Therapy* 28 (5): 385–93. https://doi.org/10.1016/0005-7967(90)90157-e.

2 **Sugar. It fires up my brain very much like a glass of wine did:**
Lustig, R., L. Schmidt, and C. Brindis (2012). The Toxic Truth About Sugar. *Nature* 482: 27–9. https://doi.org/10.1038/482027a.

4

I'm Hungry

The Sequel

Eat, drink, for tomorrow we shall die.
THE BIBLE

I've got two-thirds of this in the bag.
MY BRAIN

Let's talk about donuts.

I wrote about half of the book *Bottled* in a cute little donut shop in Manhattan, Kansas. Varsity Donuts had great coffee, lots of light, and it smelled like brown sugar. They rented out bikes and had checkerboards and tall tin ceilings. They were, in sum, my vibe. I would sit at the front window on a tall stool, order a large black coffee, and write for hours. The coffee came hot, in heavy white mugs, and I strongly feel that all coffee should be served this way. I'd work my way through edits while I drank multiple cups, and then, I would order two donuts and even more coffee. Varsity Donuts had the Strawberry Otis, an airy concoction with a tart strawberry glaze that made me gleeful. This was fitting because Varsity's slogan is "Donuts Make People Happy," and I agree. I have their t-shirt, a coffee mug, and a lot of happy memories there to prove it.

A good donut can solve a lot of problems.

But a good donut can start some problems, too.

Maybe it's the yeast. I don't know. I'm not the one to blame yeast for all my problems, but it's a main player in alcohol, so maybe it's all connected. Besides, "yeast," if you keep writing about it, sounds kind of *icky*.

After *Bottled* came out, I was the keynote at a sober writers' retreat at a writing center where I had always longed to speak. This was awesome. It was a dream realized. Set in a beautiful Arts and Crafts mansion in downtown Kansas City, Missouri, the large sunny room welcomed lots of listeners, and the whole thing was a joy for me. I invited my friend Meredith, whom I hadn't seen in ages, and having her in the front row made me feel like a rock star. Meredith has this way of leaning forward and nodding that just helps you along; she's like a therapist and groupie all in one, and I loved her for it. The whole thing was just *wonderful*.

I'm using words like "awesome" and "wonderful," which aren't the best writerly words. Writers need to show, not tell, but all I can come up with is "It was awesome." This is mainly because my memory of it is happy, all glossy and smooth. My recollection has no bumps or ridges or snaggly parts. Happiness is slippery, I guess.

One of the weirdest things that happened to me when I got sober was that I realized I wanted to drink when good things happened. This was unexpected. I figured that stressful events would trigger me, and I prepared for them to the best of my ability, but when something happy occurred? A voice inside piped up with, "Oh HO! We should totally drink at this amazing thing! If we don't, then it's like it never happened!"

If a super fun tree falls in the forest, but we didn't drink over it, did it even happen?

So, the event at The Writers' Place had been . . . amazing. It was all just so lovely that it needed a celebration, a marker, tagging it as a Really Good Memory, not to be forgotten. And that's where the donuts come in.

As I got in my car to drive home, I felt tired. My brain felt buzzy. There had been a lot of people-ing, a lot of talking. I had that weary tightness in my jaw that told me I had been smiling over my quota. I am a social introvert, which means I love people and connect deeply with them, but when I'm done? I'm done. I seriously needed to refuel.

So as I left town, I decided to stop by a local trendy donut shop and buy a half dozen for my sons. This was a kitschy joint with gigantic donuts that have become so popular in the past few years. Small children love these places. There are donuts with a mound of Captain Crunch on them, for those who wish to destroy their soft palates. There are donuts the size of salad plates, drizzled with maple syrup and bacon. The shelves were loaded with glistening donuts in Barbie colors, skewered by a Pixie Stick and a waiver. It's true. Donuts make you happy.

I bought five of the stickiest ones and one old-fashioned for myself and cheerfully carried my box out to the car. And I thought, "I'll set them up front, so I can snack on mine on the way home."

My old-fashioned buttermilk donut sat primly alongside the others, like that one girl who entered ninth grade from homeschool and wore a jean skirt every day. She was plain, but she was good.

I ate it delicately, savoring each bite. She was all simple, golden, and crispy. And I thought to myself, *Now, this is how it's done. I'm really enjoying the bite. I'm eating slowly. I'm taking in all the senses. Do I detect a bit of nutmeg? I think I do. I'm finding this to be a meaningful and intuitive moment with my pastry. This is a fully realized donut.*

I think you know where I'm going with this.

I ate all the donuts.

My weirdness around food didn't start until I was living on my own in that cute little bungalow. Before that, I can remember having abundant access to food with no rituals or hang-ups.

Well, except maybe:

1. When I was about thirteen, somebody mentioned that I had a chubby chin, and since then, my chin is a buzzkill. Like, my chin was responsible for broken relationships and possibly my entire single situation in my thirties after I'd been dumped. It's all my chin's fault.[1]

2. Once, my dad was gifted a huge chocolate bar from Nestle for his work, and we all had access to this behemoth for weeks. It was on a tray in the pantry, and as soon as you opened the door, you were hit with its sweet smell. I whittled away at that thing like a sculptor, sneaking chunks the size of my palm down to my room, so I wouldn't get the "not before dinner" lecture from my mom. There was so much joy in this. Knowing that the chocolate bar would never run out, that it was always *there*. It was euphoric. It was like Willy Wonka lived in my pantry, minus

the Oompa Loompas and their shaming. I could gnaw on chocolate whenever I wanted, as long as Mom wasn't in the kitchen. That feeling of excess seemed to answer some sort of unknown question in me that I had been asking for a long time.

3. I mirrored that type of excess when I moved into my first apartment after college. On weekends, with no plans but a movie and wine, I would first hit the grocery store. I would carefully walk the aisle, searching for just the thing that sounded enticing. Slabs of brie cheese. Large rounds of sourdough. Ben and Jerry's. Bags of sour cream and chive potato chips. Salty, sweet, and then something sour: lemon pie. Lemon pie was my favorite. All of this was for one person. I always had enough. I never ran out of flavors. The next day, hungover and stomach hurting, I would go for a super long run.

Ok, come to think of it, I think I've had food issues for a while now.

When I got in the car and started on my drive home, the donuts were an answer. In some way, I needed to know that there were always going to be donuts. Endless boxes of them, to keep me from wanting more.

Checking the GPS, I knew I would arrive home right around dinnertime. Brian would have prepared something for the boys; he was a fan of red beans and rice, and both boys loved it. I was always kind of surprised by this—the meal was spicy and consisted of two of my boys' least favorite foods. So, when Brian mentioned that he was going to prepare it for them one Sunday evening, I was skeptical. I think I said something like, "How do you ever imagine they will eat this?" which was dumb. I didn't have to cook dinner. If Brian wanted to offer them New Orleans flair to show them culture, so that they could refuse to eat it, so be it. But, as is the way with fathers, he cooked it up, absolutely destroying the kitchen in the process, and both boys acted like it was the best thing they'd ever eaten in their entire short lives.

I envisioned my return. The living room would be a mess, and two boys would look up and start asking me for things. It made me sigh a little. My trip had been for two days; I was just now starting to relax a bit.

Caregiver burnout is real. Even sober, even with all my recovery and my love for my boys, I feel it sometimes. I call it need fatigue. It's a slow burn of constant responsibility and Sisyphean tasks, and if I wasn't careful, it swung me back and forth between overcompensating as Perfect Mom and numbing out as Couch Mom. Living in such extremes only led me to exhaustion, which then, of course, led to shame. And shame, the most predictable emotion ever, used to lead right into boxed wine.

But now it was sugar. My brain didn't even have to think about it at all. My limbic system had been hardwired for so long to squelch all signals of discomfort immediately. It's the "lizard brain" that is just interested in survival, signaling fight or flight, or freeze and fear. It reacts. It freaks out. It chews without tasting. It shouts profanity. It wants what it wants.

I know the limbic system well. It was my bestie when I was drinking.[2] It's really into razzle-dazzle, and not a lot of thinking. If the limbic system were a food, it would be that fajita dish that travels through the Mexican restaurant, shutting down all conversation and making everyone rethink their dinner order.

I merged onto the highway. This portion of the trip was just endless mile markers and groups of cows. My feelings and I stared out at the cows. We all just ruminated for a bit. First of all, I wasn't super-stoked to go home. Because of this, I felt guilty. There was a huge list of things to accomplish tomorrow, a Monday, so I felt stressed about the Monday-ness of it all. And finally, at the event, a few people asked about what I was working on next, which poked at me and made me wonder if it was possible to write a book in three weeks. I had so many feelings.

And that's when the donuts happen. All six of them.

But we are not done. I've eaten the donuts and now I'm driving stickily. That's when the thinkie part of my brain enters the chat. Because I'm already feeling lousy, my thinking is equally so. This is no logical and calm post-donut analysis. These are cognitive distortions that stretch and disfigure my thoughts. They elbow in, hike up their Dockers pants, and mansplain, "Well . . . ACTUALLY, Dana . . ."

Post-donuts, my brain marches out a slew of cognitive distortions to mess with me:

1. I'm reminded about why I am a pathetic lump (labeling).

2. And that I *always* do this (over-generalization).

3. I should eat nothing but kale and lentil soup diet tomorrow (polarized thinking).

4. I will die before I'm sixty if I keep this up (catastrophizing).

It's a fun place, my brain. These wonky thoughts roll out on a conveyor belt when addiction flips the switch. They did so when I was drinking, and they still did so when I was binging. They do like a good pattern. Because I had anxiety and depression, I drank. When I drank, my anxiety and depression worsened. The same thing happened with the donuts.

Finally, all these ideas glom together to one awful, exhausted conclusion: it's not just the eating of the donuts; it's me. I'm awful. My whole self.

To be honest, I kind of think my brain can be a real asshole.

Sometimes it's just really hard being human. I mean, did my cat Steve, while lying on the floor next to his food dish, pulling pieces of kibble slowly around his large soft white belly to his mouth, ever think, "Eating while prone? *Why do I always do this? Get it together, Steve.*"

When I got home, I snuck the box to the outside trash bin, so my boys would not find out, just like I used to do with my empty wine bottles. I was half-sick, my hands were sticky, and my head hurt. But I walked inside, hugged my family, and Brian asked, on cue, "How'd it go?"

I answered, "Great! It went great! So cool! It was really fun to see Meredith, and such a great crowd!"

It was so great. It was so cool.

My words were slick. I felt numb. I couldn't grasp hold of a way to describe the day because my senses had been glazed over.

This is not the first time I have binged on food. But this was the first time that I stole donuts from my kids. Sadly, it would not be the last.

This year, for our anniversary, I made Brian his favorite peanut butter pie. This has become a yearly tradition as he seems to love it, and I cannot think of anything to buy him. The man already owns his own weather station. So, I make the pie, and then I offer them all a slice. They sit and eat. The pie is good. It's scandalously good. It's silky and chocolatey, and there are thick dollops of whipped cream. But then I watch as Henry eats three-quarters of his slice and declares himself full. He offers the rest to Brian, finishes his milk, and that's it.

I ask, "Are you feeling ok?" He looks confused. "You didn't finish your . . ." and I gesture at Brian, who is licking the plate. "Did you not like it?"

And then he says, "Nah, it's super yum. I'm just full." It's so strange.

Charlie finishes his but never asks for Slice Two. He doesn't sneak back into the kitchen later to nibble on the uneven parts of the pie, either. The pie waits in the fridge until the next day. Nobody has Breakfast Pie. At lunch, no one asks if pie can be lunch. No one inhales it at one in the morning.

It just sits there.

The boys do this kind of stuff *all the time.* We have root beer floats for movie night, and they have a root beer float. Then they stop. I always want to go back and make another one, just to be sure that I'm good and full. A backup root beer float, if you will. I don't do this because that would be bad, but I always think about doing it. My boys just slurp one down and then sit there and watch the movie, and that's it.

They do this with chocolate cake, too. They are so weird.

I know what you're thinking. Perhaps the chocolate peanut butter pie is awful, and they're pity-eating it. I can assure you that both my boys have absolutely no problem telling me if they don't like my cooking. Charlie has repeatedly asked that I never make casseroles because they are "too soft," and I have to agree: I am the queen of a mushy casserole. Henry and Charlie are too brutally honest to ever attempt pity-eating. They like the pie.

They just don't need to eat the whole pie in one sitting.

Because my boys are teenagers now, they are both emotional wrecks about twenty percent of the time. The other day, I asked one of them to help with the laundry, and he slid to the floor in a heap and announced that I was trying to kill him. So, they do have emotions. They have all the big feelings. They let those suckers fly. But they don't let the feelings hang around long enough to get attached to anything. When they were toddlers, they got mad when I didn't cut the slices of pie exactly the same size. But they never stress-ate four slices of the pie as a result.

Back in the days of my addicted drinking, when I started to realize that I might have to stop at some point, I was horrified. Divorcing alcohol would detonate my life. So, in an uneasy truce, I started toying with moderation. I tried to dabble with not drinking until 5 p.m., or only drinking wine, or only allowing myself one glass. I tried just drinking on the weekends, or only if I was out to eat. None of these things worked. Moderation simply didn't want to have anything to do with me. I tried to introduce moderation into my marriage with alcohol, and it got weirded out and left.

And then I got sober. And I was right. My life exploded. For the next year, I picked up the pieces that I needed to keep, walked away from the crater of stuff that no longer worked, and started again.

By the way, nobody survives strafing like alcoholics. We stand in the fire and we walk away. We are the phoenix. It's a glorious thing.

But "abstinence"—that total annihilation of alcohol—still mystified some folks. A few times, someone would ask, "Wait, can't you have a small glass of champagne?"

No. No, I can't. I abstain.

People don't like the word "abstinence," and I can understand that. It has a whiff of the Baptist sex talk[3] to it, and most folks don't feel comfortable with the totality of it. I get it.

But in this case, I can't touch alcohol.

Food, on the other hand . . .

Mistakes were being made.

When I first moved into my little bungalow, my dad came over to do what dads do. He wandered around and told me stuff that needed fixing. I followed him out to the backyard and found him standing, staring up at the roof on the south end of the house.

"When was the last time those were cleaned out?" He glared at the gutters.

The gutters of this house were something I had never thought about. I didn't say anything.

Dad was in a soft, short-sleeved work shirt that was so worn it was nearly transparent. He wore jeans and work boots, and his hands were on his hips, standing in the way that matched photographs of his dad, Reede. He thought about things like gutters. He was a fixer. His intensity about gutters was not, at that moment, really matching mine. This was a common occurrence.

He said to me, "Gutters, Dana. They're the most important thing. They will *destroy* foundations. *Destroy* it. And then? It's over. We're talking *thousands* of dollars."

Dad is really a downer at times.

Also, he is always right.

That fall, we had a lot of rain. And I never attended to the gutters. I just forgot about them. The gutters must have overflowed repeatedly, but I didn't really notice. What I did finally notice was that one evening, while it was pouring outside, I went down to the basement to fetch some toilet paper and saw water spurting out *through the walls*. Small jets of water, on the south end of the room, were arcing through the air and landing a good two feet out onto the cement floor. I stared at this for a moment and then reached out to place my hand on one jet of water, only to watch another jet start up to the side of it.

Homeownership can be scary.

The thing is, during Covid-19, I had started to see my sobriety like those gutters. I knew they were there. They were up there, all installed and important and in place. So, that's it, right? They protected and kept the bad stuff away. I went to meetings. I still talked about my recovery. I reached out. But probably not as often as I should, and certainly not when I was also being pelted with a lot of fear and anxiety. Storm clouds were everywhere, but I had gutters.

I didn't want to deal with the muck.

Who does?

And slowly, cracks started to appear.

Behavioral addictions are processes, instead of substances, that stimulate us, like endless internet scrolling, shopping, or gaming, until they turn into a dependency. When I speak about my alcoholism, I often refer to behavioral addictions as "sister addictions." They're *family*. The relationship can be love/hate, but it's certainly comfy. Behavioral addictions, on the rise after Covid, are largely viewed as much less harmful because they are less physiological, but they made my soul just as sick and sad and "hooked" as my alcoholism.

In my case, my behavioral addiction to food was just a long conversation I was having with myself about Want. But, you know how you can have a full-on discussion with someone and never really invest in their words? Like, the whole time you're just planning what you're going to say next? I did that with food for a long time. I chattered on about how I deserved the cupcakes and how I was fine. I threw the word "foodie" around a lot. All this eating made sense. I'd made three dishes from Julia Child's *Mastering the Art of French*

Cooking. Obviously, I was a gourmand. With all sincerity, I said things like food was my *passion.*

All of this was bullshit. I figured that out around the time my son Charlie found my stash.

The funny thing about sobriety is that it ruins binging. I was still doing it with food, but sobriety had made it not fun. "Secrets make us sick" and all that. I could hear my old friend, Mo, with his gravelly voice, brusquely telling me to snap out of it. To drown out his voice, I kept at it with loud crinkly wrappers and potato chips. Chips have a really loud volume. The salty crunching can zone me out in seconds. Or, if Brian was gone, I would stay up in my bed late at night, eating Reese's peanut butter cups that I had bought for my kids. I would keep unwrapping and eating, one after another. This led to my demise, as is the way with icky behavior. I had asked Charlie to help vacuum our bedroom, and as I was cleaning up down the hall, I heard him say, "Uh, Mom?" He came out of the room with a weird look on his face and handfuls of orange wrappers in his hands. I stared at him. And he gave me a look that withered me. "Did you eat all of these? These wrappers . . . they were falling out from under the mattress."

Feeling ashamed in front of your son is a new kind of pain.

But here is where I did something right. A couple of wrappers had fluttered to the floor, and I bent to pick them up, hiding my red face. And then I stood up, took a breath and said, "I have a problem with sugar. I'm . . . working on it."

I hadn't been working on it, really. But at that moment, right then, the work began. I had said something out loud. I don't think my son realized the importance of this because he just muttered, "You owe me about twenty of these," and went back to vacuuming.

I spoke. And then I got quiet. Defeat can do that to a person. Defeat can be good. It empties. It would eventually force me to listen to Need and to Want.

But for now, I was just broken. And all I could do was try hard not to judge this feeling by its very smooshy cover.

Notes

1 Thank you, Nora Ephron, for your book *I Feel Bad About My Neck*. I, too, feel bad about my neck.

2 The limbic system is not all bad. It keeps us alive. If we are in a catastrophe, it tells us to run. The issue is, we are so rarely in those "Help I'm being chased by a lion" scenarios anymore that sometimes the limbic system fritzes out and needs an outlet, and so one night when we are already sleep deprived we kind of snap and sit up and shout, IF YOU DON'T STOP SNORING I'M GONNA SMILL YOU at your husband because you're so tired and you started to say "kill" but then you felt bad so you substituted with "smother" and here we are. When Brian snores he does kind of sound like a lion, so I can see the connection that my poor lizard brain is trying to make. The limbic system: Not the smartest, but it means well.

3 In my teenage years, we attended a Southern Baptist church. This was so fun. The congregation was mainly old people, and my dad always joked that we needed to get there early because it took so long to file in behind all their walkers before the service started. If you are not aware of the Baptist sex talk it goes something like this: SEX IS BAD. DON'T HAVE IT. Or, if you must, get married at nineteen and jump right in, so you can be fruitful. God wants you to have *lots* of sex then. But also, there's always a whiff of sin circling around the whole thing. So, have lots of babies. But don't enjoy it. Or if you do, don't let on. So, in sum: I still have no idea what the Baptist sex talk is.

Bibliography

1 **My limbic system had been hardwired for so long to squelch all signals of discomfort immediately:**
Fuhrman, J. (2022, September 30). *Negative Effects of Sugar on the Brain*. Verywell Mind. https://tinyurl.com/37mhn8r2.

2 **Post-donuts, my brain marches out a slew of cognitive distortions to mess with me:**
Grinspoon, P. (2022, May 4). *How to Recognize and Tame Your Cognitive Distortions*. Harvard Health. https://tinyurl.com/46538k7r.

3 **Behavioral addictions, on the rise after Covid:**
Alimoradi, Z., A. Lotfi, C. Y. Lin, M. D. Griffiths, and A. H. Pakpour (2022). Estimation of Behavioral Addiction Prevalence During COVID-19 Pandemic: A Systematic Review and Meta-analysis. *Current Addiction Reports* 9 (4): 486–517. https://doi.org/10.1007/s40429-022-00435-6.

5

Vacancy

You know those old black-and-white war films of the bad guy soldiers marching and high-stepping all over the place? Well, that's menopause. I know this sounds a bit extreme. It isn't cancer. It's not Covid. But there are a lot of women out there (sober or otherwise) who have watched helplessly as menopause marched right on in and plundered their bodies and their minds, and it was having some alarming effects on my sobriety.

"Just take a seat on the table," my nurse says. "And, here's your gown." She holds out a paper towel. I'm at a doctor's appointment in late 2020, and it's the first time in a very long while that I have been in one of these rooms because we all had to cancel our appointments during the pandemic. But now, here I am, and the nurse eyes me over her mask and gives the table a little pat. I spot stirrups tucked up under the ledge of it, and I sigh. Before she leaves, she reminds me how to put on the paper towel. "Make sure the opening is in the front in an awkward way, and take a seat."

It's really not necessary to call it a *gown*, Linda.

This paper towel is, in fact:

1. Loud. It crinkles every time I move, and I'm having a hard time keeping it tucked under to protect me from the cold table. So, every time I adjust, I sound like someone is wadding me up and throwing me in the trash. Because I'm a writer, this is a metaphor.

2. Decked out in the largest and pointiest shoulders possible. It's giving 1980s power suit but without any power at all.

3. Completely unnecessary as I had been told there would be no examination today.

I lay back and stare up at the fluorescent lights. I sigh so deeply it flutters the gown. I don't want an examination. I'm here for breathing issues and fatigue and some weird nervousness, and the fact that I'm trying to keep a paper towel closed over my vagina is not helping with that. But here we are.

The part that redeems this a bit is Melissa, my doctor. I can only see her eyes over her mask, but they are kind and often crinkle into what I assume is a smile. She talks to me the entire time she is, as my husband delicately calls it, "all up in there," and I find this endearing and weird. It's ok. Likely, this is not the first vagina she has seen today. This is probably all normal for her, so she's bored and wants to ask me about my son's wrestling season. I answer with a few squeaks to help her understand that this feels awful, but doable, at the same time.

This, dear readers, is a pelvic exam. Awful, but doable. It just doesn't know how else to market itself.

For those of you reading along, wondering how a pelvic exam ties into the fact that I cannot seem to take deep breaths anymore, I wasn't sure either. Welcome to the wonderment that is menopause. Melissa finished her exam and patted my knees. "I'm gonna step out; you get dressed and then we'll talk, ok?" I was able to dramatically pull off my gown and throw it down like I was in *Grey's Anatomy*, but completely naked, which sort of helped my mood. When she knocked and entered, I was sitting there, fully dressed, and she said,

"Well, Dana, everything seems to be fine, but I'm wondering if you might be premenopausal."

And I heard, "Dana. You old."

I was fifty-one. I didn't *feel* fifty-one. It's the age that I always thought my mom was when I was a teenager. It was an impossible age; I'm more like a solid thirty-seven.

Actually, that's not true. This doctor's visit was finally happening because in the past six months, I had started to feel really lousy all the time. When I made eye contact with myself in the mirror, the woman staring back at me, with wrinkles around her neck and exhausted eyes, I guess she was starting to feel very much 51.[1] Or beyond.

It started with the breathing thing. Around three in the morning, in the darkness and quiet of a sleeping house, I would wake up, choking. My husband and dog, Rey, would be sleeping all furry and cute next to me, and I would choke awake, trying to take in air when it felt like my neck had become a closed fist. I would sit up, swing my legs over the side of the bed, and slowly try to believe that I was not dying.

Sitting there, in the darkness of a sleeping house, while contemplating why I just almost died amid all the peace and the snoring, it's a lonely moment. Then, I would get up, go to the bathroom, get a sip of water, and tell myself it was just a bad dream.

This went on for a couple of months. That's a lot of bad dreams. The thing is, if you keep thinking you're dying each time you go to sleep, then sleep loses its flavor. There is something so terrible about 3 a.m. fear. I would walk down the hall and stand at the bathroom window, staring out at the church behind our house. It's an old white church with a tall steeple, white even against the black night sky. A small circular stained glass window of an angel glows like a beacon.

Years ago, when it was 3 a.m. and I had a crying baby in my arms, I would check in with that angel. When postpartum depression had me holding a baby and also holding my breath, it felt like this. But mainly, these recent episodes reminded me of when I had been drinking, when the middle-of-the-night crazies would claw at me, and I would be at that window wondering how I could stop drinking and not die. That's what this all felt like. Despair at three am.

Not menopause felt like I was drinking again; instead, this time, I needed a detox from my own anatomy, which is pretty heavy stuff. I couldn't make sense of it. I was losing trust in my own body.

This was despair at 3 a.m. It seemed cruel.

The next morning, I would be exhausted, but there were breakfasts to be made, and laundry, and writing, and I did that thing where I wiped it down, my 3 a.m. despair, and folded it up with the kitchen towels and put it away. We were in lockdown because of Covid, and I couldn't afford to fall apart.

Instead, I decided to make the pandemic all right. My photo feed from 2020 is full of two things: pictures of my boys with our cat Steve and cookies. I baked my way through 2020. I made homemade granola and snickerdoodles. I think I even tried, once, to make yogurt in my crock pot, and we all had watery smoothies for a week and kind of hated it. Brian got Covid and spent his birthday in our downstairs office with an air mattress. We sang Happy Birthday to him outside the door, and I told him I loved him, and despair was still there, a slow, tired wail for me at every bedtime. But there were groceries to order. I no longer wiped them down and left them on the front porch because I was tired, but I thought I probably should, and I felt fear about that.

The boy's friends asked to come play and set up a Monopoly game on the front porch because if they were outside, the Covid-19 germs couldn't kill them. Right? It would be all right. Once I brought out a plate of homemade banana bread and then realized with horror that I baked it with my own hands, and hands have germs, and I might have killed someone. The banana bread was devoured before I turned back to replace it with packaged pretzels. It was the banana bread of doom. Or not, because they were fine and came back the next day and asked for some, and I said no because homemade is bad for you.

I was slowly sliding into some hardcore anxiety issues. But, wasn't everyone?

At my doctor's appointment, Melissa suggested hormone replacement therapy. She had taken a blood sample, and it "looked like I might be premenopausal. It was inconclusive." I turned it down. My sister had breast cancer in her forties. My grandmother had died from it. I had read an article somewhere that told me that HRT was bad if cancer was in my family. I didn't feel ready to have to think about menopause. I was here for the throat thing. I remember her looking at me, over her mask and plastic headgear thing, and I thought I saw concern, but who can tell with all that in the way? She told me she wanted me to come back in six months and prescribed Ambien for sleep. But ultimately, I rescheduled that appointment too because someone was sick, I think (Brian and I both had Covid twice). I moved it, along with my health, to some indefinite time in the future. I kept on wiping things down, folding things up, and putting them away.

Even before the global pandemic, doctor visits were never my priority. This was because I was raised by Jim, who was tougher than doctors. We didn't go to the doctor unless it was the last resort, and even then, there was a sense of failure. All medical issues were solved with Vicks VapoRub and gargling salt water. My son Henry has allergies, and the first time he explained his symptoms, I was reaching for a heavy mug and the hot water and salt before he finished. "Here," I slid it across the kitchen island. "Gargle with this. It will help." Watching my son try to gargle as an amateur was frustrating. He spewed water at a spot directly above the kitchen sink, and I kind of wanted to step in and help, but there's no way to help someone gargle. They have to fight through it. This was how my husband learned that using a neti pot was not waterboarding. I did tell him to tilt his head more, as the saltwater filled his head and he started slowly drowning. "What?! *gasp* Why is this . . . HOw? Where is it going? This is awful! Why would anyone? Are you trying to kill me? I can't!" he gasped and choked and sputtered, and I watched, pitilessly. Today, he is a full convert. Waterboarding beats a doctor's visit every time.

But now, at 3 a.m., I was waking up choking and gasping and craving for breath. And one night, a small miracle occurred because my husband actually heard me[2] and woke up too.

The miracle was very short-lived because he does ask a lot of questions (see above with the neti pot), and when you're dying, it's tough to take a press conference. The conversation went something like this:

Husband: Are you ok? What's going on? What is it? Why? Where? Baby, what? Why? How? When? Can I help? Can you cough, speak, or breathe? Do you know Jesus as your personal Lord and Savior? Again, can you tell me exactly *why* this is happening? And, earlier today, I misplaced my Royals baseball cap. Do you happen to know where it is?

Me: Just a moment. Let me see if I'm going to live, and then I'll get back to you.

Brian likes to fully understand every aspect of scenarios just as they come at you, and his overuse of questions in this marriage has been well documented in all of my books. A simple pat on the back would have been helpful, but instead, I had Mr. Data Collection guy in bed with me, with rumpled hair and an increasing ability to annoy me. Being annoyed while thinking you are dying is, as Brian would put it, non-value-added.

I finally slowed the gasping and whispered, "I just . . . I can't breathe." Before he started in on the second wave of questions, I held up a weary hand. "This . . . " I gestured toward my chest, " . . . has been going on for a while now. I don't know why. I just can't seem to breathe. My throat closes in on me and . . . It's awful." And I started to cry.

Brian then came in with a winning move and gathered me up in his arms, and I took one long, deep, and successful breath of air. When he's not annoying me, he calms me down.

I don't do what Brian tells me very often, but he said something along the lines of, "If you don't go to the doctor about this, there will be an 'or else' situation here," and so I did the very adult thing and finally made another appointment.

Melissa wasn't available. A male doctor with tired eyes entered the room and looked at me briefly, and we started on the same list of questions. I know this isn't his fault. I know they have to ask. But sometimes I want to say to the doctors, "Don't you guys ever read the charts? All that stuff the other docs already put into the computer—it's right THERE." We talked about the breathing thing. Again.

Doctor: So you can't breathe? In what way?

Me: I wake up choking, and I can't get air. It feels like my airway is blocked. Or I'm being strangled. I guess.

Doctor: Being strangled. Is there coughing? In what way?

Deep breath. I get it. I do. It's good that there are questions because I would probably complain if there weren't, so you can't win, Doctor. You can't. But how do I explain "in what way" that I feel like I'm dying each night?

As I try to discuss my symptoms, my brain starts to feel insecure. I'm met with two issues: One, I am suddenly convinced that the symptoms are kind of stupid, and I shouldn't have come. Or two: I can't give accurate information to all the questions because I am lousy at paying attention to my own life. When he asked me when my last period was, I snort-laughed and said, "Melissa said I'm maybe premenopausal, so who knows?" to which he said nothing and looked at the chart. I felt like a sham. I should have written this stuff down. I should have paid attention. I should have written *Auntie Flo* on the calendar like women do when they're trying to figure out their wonky bodies, but it just wasn't a priority.

I've always been like this. It's a weird trick I have when my brain feels overwhelmed or stressed. It stops paying attention to the important stuff and decides it would be a good time to watch reels where people unbox different brands of ink pens[3] and try them out.

In my twenties, I found myself independent, working, buying a couch for the first time, and trying to be a grownup. This was back when your mailbox was stuffed with credit card offers, and I decided to apply to one. It was so easy. Simple.

I used the credit card a few times at TJ Maxx and then forgot about it in a unilateral way that led me to throw away multiple bills for this card that came in the mail. Yes, I did that. In my mind, I labeled them as junk mail, barely reading the branding on the small envelopes that came monthly until one of them read "OVERDUE." By the time I finally realized the envelopes labeled *Bank of Bad Credit—Overdue Notice* might be mine, I had accrued over $1,300.00 in charges and interest.

Dad, if you're reading this right now, I'm sorry. This goes right along with a fun conversation we had about how I didn't get the oil changed in my car for over a year. Oil changes had just magically happened before that.[4]

I had been a straight-A student, right up through college. And I couldn't figure out how to pay a freaking Visa bill.

This kind of stuff haunts me. All my life, I have fought off the moniker of "Dana is kind of flaky" with honor rolls and tidy houses, but it still hung out. I think I have an allergy to overwhelm. Stress and overwhelm mean I fixate on all the outside variables in my surroundings, which means the kids, the husband. I micromanage the dog. When at-home learning ended and the kids went back to school, I would drop the boys off at the germ factory, saying things like, "Have a great day, boys! I love you! Do you have your masks? Because it's a global pandemic and people are dying! Make it a great day!" Then, I would drive home, throw in a load of laundry, and stare into the middle distance in a sort of under-caffeinated terror. After that daily stress show, pretty much anything about *me* was filed under "I'll get to that later."

Anxiety is the most common mental health disorder diagnosed today. Anxiety tells us that our daily existence, like getting the oil changed or answering a phone call, is dangerous. Oil changes are not usually dangerous, but my brain has become unable to differentiate. It's like anxiety clenches up my cranium, and I get sore and stuck and unable to move. Unable to change. Unable to say, "You know, this is upsetting, but I'm just gonna stretch a bit. Just let me . . . squeeze through here and move on."

A former student of mine is a very successful choreographer and dancer. I watch her videos on Instagram in awe. Haley moves with a fluidity that is muscled and yet soft. Her body flows and reaches in ways that fill a space. Even her stillness is movement. This is what I want my brain to look like when it's dealing with anxiety. Haley's dance adapts. It shudders and grasps and lifts. Her movements find the way. Haley's whole life, from when she was a junior sitting in my English class, waiting for the school day to be over so she could get to dance, has been centered around movement and emotion, and the relationship between the two. It's humbling, watching her.

Anxiety says there is no relationship between emotion and movement. Fear doesn't allow it.

Somewhere mixed in with all of this is my alcoholism. It's like there's an alcoholic chicken-and-egg scenario here. Did I drink because I was anxious? Or did the anxiety ask for a drink? There has been a lot of research that shows that anxiety and alcoholism are strongly related in either direction. We are anxious; we drink more. We drink more; we become more anxious. Alcoholism solves the equation both ways, and both in a horrible way.

Alcohol and my brain set up this sinister truce that I knew nothing about. Wine would work. Until it wouldn't. Alcohol would initially sedate and calm the anxious thoughts. And then, after a while, when the body succumbs and truly becomes physically addicted, there's this sickening uptick of fear with the drinking, like a nauseating carnival ride. The brain had built up a tolerance, and any sort of sedative glow had now been replaced by despair at 3 a.m. It's such a betrayal.

But now, nearly ten years sober, here I was, back at that window in the middle of the night, shaky and nauseous and triggered all over the place. Like any good alcoholic, I learned about triggers and how to anticipate them, how to get the car keys in hand, and get out of the wedding reception before the forty-year-olds start twerking. But I was not ready for *this*. I didn't know how to maneuver this at all. It sounded so ridiculous to accuse menopause of feeling like withdrawal. It's just menopause. It's *normal*. Half the world goes through this.

At 3 a.m. I knew I wasn't going to drink. My tired, sober soul still wearily waved its hand and said, "Yep. I'm here. Not gonna drink today." But that's about it. That's all I could muster.

Around this time, my body and brain decided to dial up an old stress response. I pulled down the shades a little on my life, and I got very blank.

Vacancy was comfortable. It was easy. And, it was a compromise. What mom doesn't like a good compromise? Totally shutting down was not possible. I had to get the oil changed, write an article, and figure out how to make a casserole for dinner that wasn't mushy. But vacancy meant I could do all that. I could make a list and cross things off, and just not really pay all that much attention. I would hum listlessly and stare out the kitchen window. It was like my brain had decided that movement was just a skim across the surface, not a deep dive.

My dog Rey occasionally just stands still, staring at a chair, with such fixation that I too would eye the chair, wondering if it was mean to her. The chair would be all chill, and yet Rey would continue staring at it. I sort of envied her. Alcohol used to make me feel totally vacant, but I can't anymore because I'm sober, and also, there's always somebody who needs me to drive them to baseball practice. I would watch Rey and her chair. She could stay that way for minutes, seemingly zapped out. Sometimes she would shift her gaze to me and then stare at me for weird, mournful minutes, and I would want to wave my hand in front of her or offer her a treat to snap her out of it. It was unsettling, mainly because when Rey wasn't taking what looked like a total power down with a chair, she was a large, floofy cannonball of blonde energy, burrowing into blankets on the couch or spinning after her tail. She was not brilliant, but she was action.

I asked our vet about this, because why not get concerned about your dog's weird existential vibe-outs. They kind of bothered me. Maybe she had a tumor? Looking back, I wondered if it was because I thought I had become as disconnected as a dog. But then my vet blew my theory. Wendy just laughed. "My dog does that all the time," she said. "She's actually just focusing on other sensory things, like smells and sounds, all around her." So, Rey wasn't leaving the building at all; she was just figuring out that the casserole that I had started working on was going to be delicious despite what my children might say. I envied that kind of commitment, to completely stop and take in the senses, to drift so much into smells and sounds, her surroundings, that she would stand, splayed, in frozen allegiance to them. I could learn a lot from Rey, but that won't happen until Chapter 18.

There have been studies that show that pet owners who are strongly attached to their floofy cannonballs of blonde have a higher chance of being susceptible to dissociating when stressed. Granted, I don't think I was truly dissociating. Instead, I seemed to be just stepping into a blank space daily; I guess in a dissociation-lite type of way. I don't want to downplay the seriousness of dissociative disorder. That is not my intent. (But also, as I write this, I wonder, how many of us suffer from mental health disorders, but shuffle them aside or downplay them? Why do we do that?)

My second doctor's visit was a study of overwhelm and then vacancy. He kept trying to get me to pin down my symptoms, and then he shifted gears and started asking for a timeline about periods. My answers got increasingly glum and scattered, along the lines of "I don't remember" and "Uh, maybe a year ago?" I had attempted to answer all of these specifics with Melissa, but this doctor was having none of it. I felt like a small child with each question. "You can't remember the date of your last period? Think harder. Just think *harder*, Dana." I could feel myself slowly shutting down.

The doctor did some blood tests. I waited. He came back into the room and told me I was menopausal. I nodded and said, "Yes." I was told to go on HRT. I accepted this because I was tired. He wrote the prescription. And finally, I asked,

"But the sleeping thing. The breathing. What do I do about that?" Then he turned to me and said,

"I'm going to prescribe an anti-anxiety medication for you." He was looking down, scribbling away. I took a breath.

"I'm in recovery. Can we make sure this is not something that will mess with that?"

He stopped scribbling and didn't look up, but started looking at my chart, slowly paging back and back some more. Silence.

This is the fun part. The part where you tell a stranger, "I'm sober." And there's that weird silence where they take that information and file it. It shouldn't matter to you where they file the information, or even if they just toss it out the window. It should not matter. At all. But because I had been sitting in this tiny room for over an hour now, and because our conversation previously had felt like I had been called to the principal's office, and because I didn't know this man but he was supposed to be a trusted and very personal source of help for my own body and my mind, I felt . . . small.

"In . . . recovery. Hm. So, you are in recovery." He was poring over the pages now. Does he know what I mean? Do I need to add, just to be clear, "Hey I used to drink so much wine, like boxes of the stuff because who even can bother with bottles and corks, and then I stopped because it was killing me but I'm fine now, and I'm not an awful person?"

I cleared my throat. "Yes. Sober. Since 2014." I sat up a little straighter. I tried to feel proud of that. I *was* proud of that. So why did it feel like I was throwing a wrench in this man's plan for me?

"So, that's great. I don't think Xanax—"

"Xanax? No, I don't . . . No Xanax." I pictured the Lortabs prescription after I had a C-section. I kept them for a long time after the surgery, while I was still in full-on addict mode. I kept them because maybe one day I wouldn't have wine handy, and perhaps a Lortab or two would do the trick. I eyed them every time I opened the medicine cabinet, just sitting there among the Q-tips and my eye drops. Waiting. Wreckage in my medicine cabinet. I finally disposed of those pills during my first week of recovery, feeling proud of myself and also like I wanted to scream. They were my backup plan, and I flushed them away. It frightened me. I vowed to never get started on pills because something in me knew that pills would probably kill me.

I continued on. "Besides, this is more like a breathing thing? Like . . . a choking?"

"Yes. Like a strangling. Right. Can you explain the strangling?" He had not yet looked up from his papers.

Stress shrivels the brain. It wrings out the prefrontal cortex, which is sort of the more sophisticated part of the brain, the one wearing the power suit that makes big important decisions and does all the adulting. Stress powers it down, and instead, my lizard brain, the amygdala, gets all overstimulated, and I feel blank rage when one of my sons named "Not Me" spills Ovaltine on the kitchen counter[5]. Rage at nine in the morning is inappropriate, and so after it splutters all over, the brain dials down to an eerie emptiness. My brain leaves my brain. I become vacant and alone, and very quiet. By the end of my visit with this doctor, I was mutely nodding. I couldn't seem to think straight, and I couldn't seem to care. I was vacant.

I took the prescription for the Xanax. And I left.

Notes

1. There is nothing wrong with the number 51. But as one who still, occasionally, wonders how in the world the universe decided I was mature enough to even get married and have kids, and whose husband is starting to get mailers from the AARP, it can be unsettling. I still, on some days, feel 18. Which simply means there are days when it's like I don't have enough information yet to be fully locked in. I'm still processing. I am that wheel of annoyance on the computer that just doesn't want to open the document yet. Someday, I guess, I'll feel 51. Until then, I'll keep slowly spinning.

2. Brian: Sleeping
Someone drops a piano outside our door: BLAM
Brian: Sleeping

3. Give me a Bic Cristal black medium ballpoint. It has just the right tug and glide, and yes this is a thing. I am not a fan of gel pens, even though everyone raves about them, although I do like a black Sharpie S-gel, but they go dry too quickly. Looking for the best writing pencil? Try a Palomino Golden Bear #2, the blue ones.

4. Other magical things that happened before full-on adulting: Gutters and college payments.

5. It is statistically proven that if a drink stands alone in a room and then a son enters that room, the drink has a 94.6 percent chance of being spilled. Add the variable of powdery mix-ins and we're at 99.9 percent. Also, the cleaning of the spillage is inversely proportional to the size of the spillage. All moms know this. It's science.

Bibliography

1. **Menopause felt like I was drinking again:**
   Stines, PsyD, Sharie (2018, August 31). "When Stress Is Toxic: Your Brain and Stress Response." *GoodTherapy.org Therapy Blog.* https://www.goodtherapy.org/blog/when-stress-is-toxic-your-brain-and-stress-response-0831185.

2. **Anxiety is the most common mental health disorder diagnosed today:**
   Šimić, Goran, Mladenka Tkalčić, Vana Vukić, Damir Mulc, Ena Španić, Marina Šagud, Francisco E. Olucha-Bordonau, Mario Vukšić, and Patrick R. Hof (2021). Understanding Emotions: Origins and Roles of the Amygdala. *Biomolecules* 11 (6): 823. https://doi.org/10.3390%2Fbiom11060823.

3. **Did I drink because I was anxious? Or did the anxiety ask for a drink?**
   Hassan, Ahmed N. (2018). "Patients with Alcohol Use Disorder Co-Occurring with Depression and Anxiety Symptoms: Diagnostic and Treatment Initiation Recommendations. *The Journal of Clinical Psychiatry* 79 (1): 69–71. https://doi.org/10.4088/jcp.17ac11999.

4. **There have been studies that show that pet owners who have a really strong attachment:**
   Brown, Ellen, and Aaron Katcher (2001). "Pet Attachment and Dissociation." *Society & Animals* 9: 1. https://www.animalsandsociety.org/wp-content/uploads/2015/11/brown1.pdf.

5. **Stress shrivels the brain:**
   Hathaway, Bill (2012, January 9). "Even in the Healthy, Stress Causes Brain to Shrink, Yale Study Shows." YaleNews. https://news.yale.edu/2012/01/09/even-healthy-stress-causes-brain-shrink-yale-study-shows

6

Risk

And now I am holding a prescription for Xanax, and I am having a conversation with my inner alcoholic. I call her Britney. She spells it with a little heart above the "i" and she is a sociopath.

There are times when my alcoholism likes to bargain. Even after years of sobriety, there can still be a tiny voice that says things like, "Well, this will be alright. It's not going to mess you up. In fact, it might fix everything. C'MON, Dana." There's a longing there, sometimes, for such a fix because that's what alcohol did for a while, in a screwed-up, totalitarian way.

True, you know you can't drink. But this isn't drinking. And your doctor prescribed it. I'm sure lots of people take this, and they're in recovery, and they're fine. Totally fine. So, you could be one of those people. This might make you feel better. Or, maybe it's just going to make you feel floaty, and that is going to make you feel *better*.

Perhaps someone is reading this who takes Xanax in a normal way, and I need you to know two things:

1. Good. Medication is made to help us. It's your journey.
2. My journey has addiction in it. It's not just a detour. It's a frontage road, always running parallel and offering multiple exits. Some of those exits are permanent. So, I am envious of you, just a little. It's complicated.

My inner alcoholic and I had quite a bit of back and forth after my appointment, and then there was a long silence from both of us. Finally, Britney said, "The Xanax will make you feel buzzed. Don't you remember?"

And so, here we are.

Imagine having a dinner party where you invite all your addictions and maladaptive coping skills and weird little hang-ups [1]. Just imagine it. Nothing says dinner party like slowly building dread, yet that's where I was, sitting at the head of the dysfunctional table. We were a little crowded, but we made it work.

At the far end of the table is Britney, aka alcoholism. This is the true asshole of the bunch. She doesn't have a drink in front of her, which is totally ticking her off, but she's there. The thing is, when you get sober, alcoholism is a permanent fixture, even if you would prefer it not to be. I would like to say I got sober like it was a big one-time event, and when I did so, my addictions packed up and left, like vacating a grungy motel room in my mind, forever gone. But instead, they are still in that motel room, waiting. It's a motel room that I can go back to any time I like. Knowing this helps keep me sober. The motel room from hell is a farther walk now, but it's still there. It's a forever motel room.

Next to Alcoholism is Disordered Eating. She's been around almost as long as the drinking thing. She's especially antsy because it's a dinner party, so food is coming and abstinence is kind of off the table.[2] She's fun. She talks about salads a lot.

We have Social Anxiety, but she's already upstairs looking for cats. She thinks we are talking about her behind her back, but we have enough going on.

Generalized Anxiety is here. She's super chatty and likes to make a lot of jokes. She doesn't eat much because she doesn't want to get salad dressing on her face. One time, she had a dab of salad dressing on the corner of her mouth, and she forever remembers this as the Salad Dressing Event. It makes her very careful now. Everyone knows that being very careful with a salad just makes it not happen at all because salads don't do well with all that pressure. As the evening progresses, she'll slowly get quieter and then . . . silent. No one will know when she leaves.

There's Depression. She is also jovial and fun and totally the life of the party. She's a blast. On the drive home, she will completely detach. She won't understand at all why she hates stuff like this. At some dinner parties, this doesn't happen, and then she thinks she's cured. And then it happens again, and she hates her brain. Hates it. It makes her stomach hurt.

Perfectionism will also be here. Her outfit is adorable, and she feels fat in it. Always. She will look around a lot, comparing her own mind with the minds of others. She probably hated that hotel room the most because ick, but she's one of the main reasons I went back there in 2014.[3]

Guilt somehow manages to sidle in because doesn't she always? She keeps carrying the prescription for Xanax around in her bag. She hasn't filled it yet, and she knows she'll feel massive guilt either way. She's a total downer.

There is one final guest at the table that I haven't seen in a long time. She has a lot of audacity, but she came bearing house gifts and an offer to help clean up when we're done. Codependency, my old bestie from my twenties, cuddles up to Brian and confuses the crap out of him. She is tricky. There's a lot of neediness, but it's paired with a heavy helping of narcissistic expectations, and Brian cannot figure her out. That's ok. I can't either. Basically, Miss Codependent comes with years and years of strings attached. Oh, what a tangled web we weave.

It's crowded. There's jostling of plates and weird conversations, and occasionally a mournful Rey wanders in and stares vacantly at us, then shudders and trips over a string on her way out.

Menopause sent the invite. She's at the head of the table and she's hot. No, like, literally; she's burning up. She can't remember things and feels nauseous and starving at the same time. Nobody really likes her, especially her husband, but it's normal. It's fine. It's *just* menopause.

The thing is, menopause is serving up the same dining experience that alcohol did so long ago. That's why there are so many at this table.

Research on women, addiction, and menopause is difficult to find. We're still being excluded from clinical trials and medical research of all types, and in nearly 99 percent of studies on aging, menopause is disregarded. Why? Are we just that difficult?[4] Menopause can have a negative influence on mental health disorders, namely anxiety and depression, and those were the main two reasons I abused alcohol. Anxiety started it all. It's the trickiest player in the mix because not only did it offer itself up as a catalyst for drinking, but it hung around and became the consequence. It was the mother and the offspring, and yes, that is just as icky and dysfunctional as it sounds.

Hormone fluctuations associated with menopause cause so many symptoms that their maladies are longer than even most WebMD home hypochondriacs are willing to deal with. Here's a smattering:

- anxiety
- irritability
- changes in skin conditions, including dryness or an increase in oiliness and the onset of adult acne
- insomnia
- discomfort during sex
- feelings of loss of self
- hair loss or thinning
- migraines
- hot flushes of skin and body
- increase in facial hair
- joint stiffness
- loss of self-confidence
- nausea
- night sweats
- heart palpitations
- problems with memory, concentration, and "brain fog"
- recurring UTIs
- incontinence
- reduced libido; sex problems
- tinnitus
- vaginal dryness and pain
- osteoporosis
- heart disease
- suicidal ideation[5]

I mean . . . but who's counting?[6]

Estrogen drops, and stress, and depression increase. Loss of sleep. Loss of self. Progesterone is linked to helping reduce the urge to drink—it drops, too. The safety is off. Hormones, the communicative transmitters in the brain, fritz out. They send wonky messages or stop messaging altogether.

Oh, and did I mention? Menopause can last up to fourteen *years*.

This dinner party wasn't going to end anytime soon, which is unacceptable for an introvert like me. There's always a polite time to leave, but instead, I had all these bad coping strategies and behavioral addictions that were cropping up, trying to fill in the gaps. I was trying to cope as best as my brain knew how. But there was one process addiction in there that surprised me with its return and its effectiveness: Risk.

Of all the process addictions, gambling is considered one of the most common. Additionally, it's often associated with people who have alcohol use disorders. When my brother died from alcoholism, it took my parents weeks to clean out his ravaged home. The process had been heartbreaking. Amid the sweet memories of his past and the aching reminders of who Chris was, Mom and Dad found more tragedy. He had an online gambling addiction, resulting in thousands of dollars of debt. I remember feeling shocked; Chris was good with money. We all were. Our family prided itself on thrift and hard work, and always buying everything on sale. Our family motto was "That's too expensive," and I knew Chris followed that protocol. Or I thought he did. And I can remember thinking, "How could he let it get that bad?"

My version of "bad" was just as risky; it just didn't involve money. I once lost twenty dollars within five seconds at a slot machine, and that, paired with the carpets in all casinos, kind of turned me off to the cash gambling thing. Instead, I was willing to risk everything for love.

This sounds like an 1980s song. It doesn't seem so bad. It's kinda sexy and there's more of those big feelings and big hair and synthesizers.

Here's what codependency really means:

When I was twenty-six, I was in love with a man who was not quite as in love with me. He was tall and kind and really unequipped to provide me with the guarantee that we would be together forever, but I hung on like a barnacle. Ryan rode bikes. He entered numerous races that I attended for hours, watching for him at the finish line and feeling like one of those women in the Tour de France with their bouquets of flowers and yellow dresses. We watched the real Tour at three in the morning because this was before streaming. And of course, I started riding too because that's what you do as a major league codependent player. You train, and you do drills, and you wait for a big day when you can dazzle. We were awfully cute, me in my early years of teaching and Ryan in his early years of art school.

Oh, and our relationship was centered around drinking.

He was my favorite person on the whole planet. I was probably in his top ten. We tried to be balanced, and by that, I mean I literally did everything possible to keep him interested. It was tiring, but I had more energy then.

We did a lot of things at night. One involved a cruiser pub crawl in Lawrence, Kansas, in the winter because heavy drinking, bikes, and frozen darkness are fun. It's cool. He was cool. I kept up.

I mean, literally. I kept up. His gang was a bunch of hardcore cyclists who did mountain biking and wheelies and liked marijuana a lot. There were a lot of tattoos, and this was before tattoos became a part of the wardrobe for thirty-somethings. I was not a good cyclist, but that night I kept drinking beer because everyone else was (you don't ask for a nice glass of white wine at a pub crawl when the crawlers have names like Roadie and say "derailleur" a lot.)

And then, it started sleeting.

I remember thinking, "Well, now it will get canceled and I can go to bed," but they all left the bar to get to the next one with absolutely no change in enthusiasm. One guy who looked just like Flea from the Red Hot Chili Peppers skidded by, only wearing his bike shoes. And Ryan hopped on his bike and looked at me as if to say, *This is your time to dazzle, Dana.*

Dana is a lot of things, but I'm not a risk-taker in a biking-in-the-sleet kind of way, so I can't really explain what happened next. I did drink alcoholically for years, so I understand peril. My version of risk is to hold onto men with the tenacity of a drug addict looking for a fix.

That night, I took my Trek on a downhill incline that was so steep that a pile of bikes and bodies were strewn at the bottom. I had stopped at the top and eyed the carnage below, and horrifically, Ryan and all of his friends had started cheering me on. This was not an opportunity for me to shake my head and back away, saying something like, "I hate this bike and everything it stands for." This was the time to be scrappy, so with a shaky inhale, I pushed myself over the edge, along with any sense of self.

I don't know how I managed to make it to the bottom without dying, but somehow I did. Ryan crowed and looked proud, and I thought that would be enough. About six years later, when he finally broke up with me, this downhill slalom should have been enough. I should have been able to yell, "YOU CAN'T BREAK UP WITH ME. I RODE MY BIKE DOWN THAT HILL," and he would nod and say, "Oh yeah. Ok, never mind. You rock." It should have been the thing that proved our forever bond because that's just how messed up our relationship was. But it didn't.

I learned absolutely nothing from this. During my first year of marriage, my codependent slaloms with Brian revved up because we were legally stuck with each other. The stakes were even higher. I didn't ride bikes for Brian; I did something far nuttier. I decided Brian would never get mad at me for anything.

Honestly, I would have preferred the cliff-diving bike thing, but this was the brand of risk I was dealing with in my marriage. It was a lot harder.

It continued with babies. Babies cry, you know. That means they're mad at you. And if codependency still looms, that's rough. I wanted to fix the babies and make them happy all the time. Sometimes babies don't do that.

When I got sober, I tackled codependency. Like, I *really* tackled it. I started feeling all my feelings and I got pissed off all the time. Brian was the nearest target, so I shouted, "No!" at him a lot. I didn't worry about happiness because all I was doing was trying to survive, and happiness didn't seem so important when you're just trying to stay sober an hour at a time. Then, as is the way with recovery, miracles started to happen. If a relationship is meant to be, recovery helps it through. With Brian and me, first, it got bad, and then it got *really* bad, and then it started to settle down. We began talking about our feelings in a way that makes sense.

I started making boundaries, going to meetings, and then making *more* boundaries. I started understanding my whole self in relation to others. I didn't have to be this glommed-on amoeba that clutched at my family with fear and trembling like a jello salad with a dual diagnosis. Instead, I could take on life on life's terms, and we would all live happily ever after.

Enter menopause.

What seemed to be happening now was a weird mashup of Dana slipping back into people-pleasing and self-erasing behaviors, followed up by an encore of misdirected rage. This is, as most therapists would call it, "troubling behavior."

I like to refer to it as "Fear and Loathing in Las Dana."

I had two sons who were in the middle-school years, so hormones were zinging all over that house. I would find a kid fritzing out over a missing homework assignment ("I SWEAR I put it RIGHT HERE MOM! Who moved it? WHY are PEOPLE always MOVING my THINGS?") and then he would shove a pile of papers off onto a chair while searching, to which I *might* drily mention that he had just moved someone *else's* things, which was a totally poor parenting move.

I would then feel guilty and throw myself into a search party for a crumpled math assignment[7] knowing that if I could just find it, my son and my heart would stop freaking out. My mental state was playing roulette with whoever wanted to roll the dice with me. I lost constantly. Other people's needs, real or imagined, trumped me every time.

Codependency told me: If I put all my chips down on this one thing that I can fix, it will fix it ALL. My heart. My mind. All of it. So, I'll risk it.

And then, codependency got quiet and then whispered: And if I don't fix it, people will leave.

And a pandemic and menopause said: NO ONE IS LEAVING. WE ARE LITERALLY STUCK HERE.

Alcoholics have a known aversion to uncertainty, and I think my codependency was born out of an attempt to manage this. And, during a pandemic and dealing with the under-researched and overly placated symptoms of menopause, I wasn't feeling certain about much of anything. What I was doing was going for the quick fix that promised a quick reward. It might not be a stable one or a healthy one, but it was quick and it was here. I parented badly. I stopped trying to help my child through bad behavior with discipline and reason; I fixed it for them. I also marriage-ed badly. I went all in with keeping the peace with my boundaries as bargaining chips. I coped. I tried to stay connected to my people, which was one of the best ways for people in recovery to handle the isolation of the pandemic. I had good intentions, but

I did it badly. Connection mutated into codependency. I did the best I could at the time.

Living in all of this, there was my little dog Hosmer. He was older and crankier, not as prone to vacancy as our darling blonde doggie, Rey. He was more inclined toward trembling or growling and following me into every room.

I have to admit that I had stopped noticing Hosmer as much, as the other issues in the household seemed more important than a constant brown shadow that followed me into the bathroom every time. You start to just expect it after a while, the brown shadow in the bathroom thing. Until one day, it's not there.

I was in the downstairs bathroom, you see, and Hosmer was still upstairs. This was unusual. My descent of the stairs was always followed by his thunking tap dance right behind me. But lately, he had been moving a little bit more slowly, a bit more cautiously, and I just figured it was taking him a bit longer to arrive at the bathroom door, tail wagging, much relieved to see that I had not abandoned him after all.

And then I heard a soft doggy wail and a sickening series of thumps, and I knew. Hosmer had fallen down our stairs. By the time I reached him, he was upright again and breathing hard. His tail was low, and so was his head, but when he saw me, he lifted it slowly, and his tail wagged twice. I knelt in front of him, cupped his soft ears and face in my hands, and looked at him. His eyes were cloudy, and his little muzzle was gray. I hadn't really seen this. I mean, I knew he was getting along, but all of a sudden, Hosmer was old. He slowly sat back on his haunches, but one paw slid out beneath him, and he struggled up again. He was old.

But still, he must follow me everywhere. All of a sudden, I became very aware of how many times I walked up and down our stairs in our big old house. I became aware of how high our bed must feel and how slippery the tiles were in the kitchen. I started to listen for and sort of dread the soft click of claws on the wood floor behind me. He was my shadow, but sometimes so slowly that I would just meet him in the middle and stop and stroke his soft ears. His cloudy eyes would search for me everywhere, and I started to play that fun bargaining game of when I should call our veterinarian.

Hosmer was just always *there*. Always following with short stubby legs and tired-out tenacity. He loved to sleep on our bed, and when I would finally get into it and surround myself with my pillows and a good book, he would circle about seven times and then flop with a small grunt of pleasure and relief. "She's finally stopped moving," he would think. "I can rest up for the next shift." And it would start all over again the following day.

Now, I begged him to rest. I would load his bed up with peanut butter treats and blankets, and his favorite squeaky hot dog. It didn't matter. He would creakily get to his feet every time I moved, and I would curse myself for carrying laundry upstairs. Occasionally, I would get frustrated and say, "No! Stay! STAY!" but his pitiful expression would only work me up more, and I would turn away. There would be a short silence, and then I would hear it. Those softly clicking toenails.

It was awful.

That's codependency. You follow and follow, and you follow. Even when it hurts. And it finally makes you fall.

Of course, I didn't know any of this. I was gambling it all away. Gamblers often don't even know they have a problem. Only about ten percent seek help for it, and researchers are not sure why those numbers are so low. The stigma attached to gambling problems has a part to play, which makes sense when you think back to my judgmental attitude toward Chris's debts.

The stigma of codependency also stings. If I sought help for it, I think my reasoning would have sounded something like this: I just need people to love me no matter what.

Who wants to admit to that?

So here we are back at that awful dinner party. For about a three-year period, these dinner guests had been mingling, arguing, and making more and more of a mess in my life. Perfectionism kept me from admitting it. Anxiety made me put off any sort of appointment. And codependency just made me focus on my children and my husband instead of myself.

Oh, and depression. Depression just told me nothing would ever change, no matter how I tried.

In March of 2021, the CDC gave the ok for vaccinated people to rejoin the world, even without masks. But, folks felt weird about it. Instead of shouting hurrah and slingshotting their masks into the nearest bin, people were tentative and highly anxious about breaching the outside, to "normal" living again. It felt scary. Clinicians have a name for it: Cave Syndrome. And it makes sense. It is dark and quiet here, and there's a lot of lying around, eating high-calorie foods that kept me squishy.

So, I made no move for change. I had suffered weight changes and sleep disturbances. I gained a lot of weight around 2020. Because I was ashamed and felt, literally, sick and tired all the time, I didn't want to be around people. It felt scary and weird, and also, I felt so markedly different. I knew I looked different. When friends would see me, perhaps at the store buying more donuts, I imagined they would be shocked by my appearance. I felt like lugging around this body and this brain was nothing but a burden.

This means, if I'm really really honest, that I didn't much want to be in a cave, or out of a cave, at all. I didn't want to be anywhere anymore.

I really really needed help.

Postscript: I called our vet that week, the week he fell. My boy was in pain. Our vet Molly came to our house, and I held Hosmer in my arms and whispered to him all along his way about what a good boy he was. And he was. Hosmer really was a very, very good boy.

Notes

1. I know some of you are saying, "Why even do that?" Dinner parties are for fun! But remember back to your last dysfunctional Thanksgiving dinner and that one uncle who wants to talk about chemtrails, and all those cousins who kept trying to ride the dog, and your one niece that you kind of like has decided she is vegan yesterday and turkey is murder, and you know. We love them, and they're invited, and it's a big mess.

    Also, Mom and Dad, this chapter is NOT about our Thanksgivings, ok? They are wonderful and I love them. Especially the oyster dressing and the part where we talk about gratitude. Perhaps not in that order.

2. Yes you saw what I did there, right? #pulitzer

3. I wrote a whole book about this. It's called *How to Be Perfect Like Me* and this sounds like a plug for you to read it. You don't have to. Or you can just check it out at the library if you like. And now I am pretty sure Socially Awkward should be a guest at that dining table because that's exactly what this is.

4. I know that my husband will read this book, and this is the portion where he might blink a lot, attempt to say something, and then back slowly away. Thank you, husband, for your service.

5   Female suicides are highest in the age ranges from forty-five to sixty-four years old. Studies are now linking menopausal symptoms to high rates of suicides but there is not enough research yet.

6   The latest research shows thirty-four symptoms. But since nobody really wants to research menopause because it's really hard, nobody is sure.

7   It's in the pile in the chair. It's always in the pile in the chair.

Bibliography

1   **We're still being excluded from clinical trials and medical research of all types:**
Blakemore, Erin (2022, June 27). Women Are Still Underrepresented in Clinical Trials. *Washington Post*. https://www.washingtonpost.com/health/2022/06/27/underrepresentation-women-clinical-trials/.

2   **. . . in nearly 99% of studies on aging, menopause is disregarded:**
Walsh, Jennifer (2024, January 10). How Gaps in Research Lead to Gaps in Care for Aging Women. *Harvard Medical School*. https://tinyurl.com/mwx5hu3x.

3   **Menopause can have a negative influence on mental health disorders:**
Alblooshi, Salama, Mark Taylor, and Neeraj Gill (2023). Does Menopause Elevate the Risk for Developing Depression and Anxiety? Results from a Systematic Review. *Australasian Psychiatry* 31 (2): 103985622311654. https://doi.org/10.1177/10398562231165439.

4   **Hormone fluctuations associated with menopause cause so many symptoms:**
NDFW (2020, December 18). Menopause and Addiction: How Your Hormones Play a Role. https://www.newdirectionsforwomen.org/menopause-and-addiction-how-your-hormones-play-a-role/.

5   **Here's a smattering:**
Nadeem, Dr. Hamza (2023, February 23). What Are the 34 Symptoms of Menopause? Revive Research Institute, LLC. https://www.reviveresearch.org/blog/what-are-the-34-symptoms-of-menopause/.

6   **Menopause can last up to fourteen *years*:**
National Institute on Aging (2021). "What Is Menopause?" September 30. https://tinyurl.com/2uahaxn2.

7   **Of all the process addictions, gambling is considered one of the most common:**
Caron Treatment Centers (n.d.). Process Addiction Statistics & Demographics. https://www.caron.org/addiction-101/process-addictions/statistics-demographics.

8   **It's often associated with people who have alcohol use disorders:**
Grant, Jon E., Matt G. Kushner, and Suck Won Kim (2002). Pathological Gambling and Alcohol Use Disorder. *Alcohol Research & Health* 26 (2): 143–50. https://www.ncbi.nlm.nih.gov/pmc/articles/PMC6683819/.

9   **Alcoholics have a known aversion to uncertainty:**
Gorka, Stephanie M., Lynne Lieberman, K. Luan Phan, and Stewart A. Shankman (2016). Association between Problematic Alcohol Use and Reactivity to Uncertain

Threat in Two Independent Samples. *Drug and Alcohol Dependence* 164 (164): 89–96. https://doi.org/10.1016/j.drugalcdep.2016.04.034.
10 **I tried to stay connected to my people:**
University of Iowa College of Public Health (2023, April 24). Researchers Study How People in Recovery from Alcohol Problems Coped during the Covid-19 Pandemic. *Iowa College of Public Health.* https://tinyurl.com/yk374sxv.
11 **Gamblers often don't even know they have a problem:**
Whelan, James P. (2023, February 8). Millions of Americans Are Problem Gamblers – so Why Do so Few People Ever Seek Treatment? The Conversation. https://tinyurl.com/tv93p9m9.
12 **Clinicians have a name for it: Cave Syndrome:**
Newsome, Melba (2021, May 3). "Cave Syndrome" Keeps the Vaccinated in Social Isolation. Scientific American. https://www.scientificamerican.com/article/cave-syndrome-keeps-the-vaccinated-in-social-isolation1/.

Part II

Recovery

7

Marriage Is What Brings Us Together Today

> *Reader, I married him.*
> JANE EYRE

Brian and I are at a wedding. Note: This is a Scottish wedding, so it has kilts. There are so many hairy legs at this thing, and beards. There's just a lot of hair, in general. I have been sober for four years. I am wearing a cute Betsy Johnson dress with red cherries, and I think I bought red heels for the occasion. It's going to be a party, and I need the shoes to match.

Scots like to drink, did you know? Or at least this group did. There were a lot of very elaborate mustaches that twist and turn, and tattoos that did the same. As the reception continued, I watched as people got progressively more inebriated. My husband, a normie, loves whiskey. It is one of his favorite drinks, and once, when I was still actively in my addiction, he took me to a Scotch tasting because he was interested in things like "levels of peat" and "hints of vanilla," and I was interested in getting drunk in a sophisticated way.

As we sat at the table and the noise level slowly increased because of alcohol, I looked at my husband. He was handsome in his shirt and tie, and carefully pressed Dockers. He did not have a kilt, and for this, I was truly sad. This would have been the time for it, and Brian has extraordinary calf muscles. He was downing pizza because the newly married couple felt that most folks would appreciate a pizza bar more than a chicken breast and limp asparagus. Also, everybody was getting soused, and pizza pairs well.

Brian was not soused. We had this thing that we did where Brian didn't drink when Dana was lurking about, and then he would repeatedly promise it didn't bother him.

I had to think it bothered him. This was 2018. We'd been married for twelve years. I'd been sober for four. He had made promises to me for all of those years, and the words that come out of Brian's mouth are startlingly true. He's not a liar. He's a lot of other things, but deception is not in his nature. There is an obvious reason: he's just a simple man with a lot of goodness in him. And his bad behavior tends to be the kind of "out there" type with no attempt at covering it up. I fold up my anger and store it away in a drawer labeled "seething resentments that will surface at weird times." Brian's all about being out of the drawer.

There is another reason why he doesn't lie: he's my foil, and I am literally married to a literary term. My God, the irony.[1]

Brian kept eating pizza, great big gooey slabs of the stuff, and I looked at him with a kind of wonder. We didn't know many people at this wedding. My shoes were beginning to hurt. But yet, I was having a pretty good time, and Brian had pizza and rockabilly music, so he was in wedding heaven. When he finished eating, he waited a moment and then said, "You wanna dance?" I let him spin me out on the floor with his two swing dance moves he learned back when he was single. Swing dance lessons were endlessly offered to single people at his church to make them more marketable. I preferred the slow dance, circa 1985, where we just sort of rocked back and forth and I could lean on him because my feet hurt, but still. We zipped around. It was fun.

About an hour later, I pulled out my "How to be married to a normie when you are in recovery" move and eyed him over the music and the noise, and the whiskey. I gave him our secret signal that informed him it was time for this sober girl to head out.

This is my secret signal: I look at him and say, "I want to leave."

He smiled and said, "I was wondering how long you would last."

We left, pocketing our wedding favors that were, I think, tiny bottles of Scotch. I gave mine to Brian, and we drove home in comfortable silence. Just to be sure, though, I circled back to my neuroses. "You like whiskey, and I am sorry."

He answered yes and then said, "But it's no problem, my lady," which was cringy, but also I love him, so it was fine. I guess that's the bargain. He doesn't drink around me, and I have to deal with cringe.

This is what recovery mixed in with a relationship looks like. I try hard to say, out loud, the things that might be challenging in social situations. I told Brian long ago about recovery strategies, such as taking my own car and leaving early at a point when, for some, the party is just getting started. To be honest, some of this might fit in the slot of "Is it alcoholism, or am I just an introvert?" But getting sober meant I needed to get honest about that too (I had no idea I was an introvert until around the same time I got sober. This is so weird, right? What a coincidence).

I also have to be honest and tell Brian that sometimes I wish, just for a minute, a teeny tiny minute, that I could be that person who goes to a wedding and drinks, and it is all ok. And then he says, "No, you don't. You know it wouldn't be ok. And that's ok. This is better." I tut at him and say, "I know Brian, geez," and inside I smile and hunker into him, but on the outside I'm probably folding laundry. And that's what married couples do. We hunker into each other on the inside because we are honest and comfortable, and we know the drill, and there's always laundry now.

So, that's our marriage + alcoholism.

But... What about a pandemic + marriage + alcoholism?

Or, even better, pandemic + menopause + marriage + alcoholism?

Math was never my strong suit.

A couple of weeks into lockdown, Brian had set up his work-from-home office downstairs. The boys had their space in the living room, and I floated around from room to room, trying to find my own space to write. I had a lovely office upstairs, but it was tucked up far away from both boys and their school, and also, it was a *pandemic*. I couldn't come up with any writing ideas at all, and was suffering from the same sort of manic "Let's write ALL the things" then feeling guilty because I couldn't seem to find a focus, or a way to start, or a glimmer of inspiration.

Instead, I made snacks. So. Many. Snacks.

At about 6 p.m., Brian would come tentatively out of his office as if he was checking for his shadow, and the house would breathe a sigh of relief. It was just kind of better when he was around. We would eat even more food at this point under the disguise of "dinner," but I'd been feeding them so much at this point, who's keeping track?

And we would do the same thing the next day. And I sank slowly into depression and tried not to. What I didn't know at the time was that I was also premenopausal. Cue the ominous music.

This is when being married can be tough. Depression isn't some sort of visual malady. I wasn't limping around with my leg in a cast, which honestly might have been a freaking delight because maybe then they could all get their own snacks. I got quiet. Brian didn't really notice this until he came out of his hole one afternoon for another snack, and he found me crying while mixing some cake batter.

Here is some more math. At that moment, I was looking for a way to explain how I was feeling, causing his response to somehow make me feel better. But the probability of this happening is only about 33 percent. The rest of the time, it's just one messed-up human relying on another messed-up human to fix her, and everybody misses the mark. When we first got married, I would try to explain to him how "sometimes I just feel really low," and he would tilt his head and say, "Why?" and then I was not only depressed but irritated. I couldn't explain WHY I was depressed. It wasn't situational. It just was this thing that hunkered down in my life and made me feel like everything was impossible. Brian would then fire off a list of things I should try, and I would hate him. So, after a while, I stopped trying to explain. I didn't want to be told about gratitude, because I might kill him, so I avoided the conversation altogether.

But that afternoon, we made a decision together. It started with me telling him how bad this had become and the appointments with Andrea. I said, "I need to give you a signal. Like, some sort of code when this is happening. Maybe I can just text it to you and you can know." He nodded.

"That way, you can just be aware." His mouth opened, and I held my hand up. "And you don't have to tell me anything. You just need to know."

The code was "bad brain" and yes, I realize—I should not be shaming my brain, but it's alliterative, and it stuck. I would have gone for Winston

Churchill's figurative "black dog" of depression, but I was afraid Brian would forget and think I was adopting another puppy.[2]

This did not fix it. But it helped. And that sums up my marriage right there.

I got sober when we were in year six of marriage. Some would say that sobriety would make the marriage smaller and more constrained, and at the beginning, I'm sure it did in a way. For the first year of sobriety, there were lots of borders being drawn. I had to figure out my yesses and my no's. There was a lot of reworking of my own life and my expectations in sober living, and Brian had to adjust to this new, kind of baby Dana, figuring it all out and squalling at some points. Nobody really signs up for a marriage when, six years into it, a refurbished wife shows up, one who is just now learning how to feel her feelings and live with her insides matching her outsides. It's a lot. It's hard. There's all this communicating that has to be done. And praying. And detaching. And adjusting. And accepting.[3]

When I got sober, there was the first big fight that we had, and then I realized that, oh, this is terrifying because it's not fueled with alcohol, so it's a *real* argument. It's pretty bad, which makes me wonder, will we make it? Is this going to work? How do we fight now?

And there's sober sex, which the first time around just kind of shocked me with all the things I didn't pay any attention to before. There are so many details.

There are conversations about the really hard things, like money or illness, and I thought, "Oh yeah, this is fear without alcohol, and he's not going to be able to fix that either. How do I do this?"

Also, we've been married for a long time, and there's boredom and a conversation you have with yourself about passion. I glance over and he's eating chicken wings like a piranha with sauce all over its gills, and I think, *How do I do passion now with a piranha that has sauce all over it?*

There's menopause, which ushered in a whole new level of rage—the hormonal kind—which isn't good for any type of relationship. Since Brian is married to me, he's all up against me in such a personal way; therefore, he is often in the way of that rage.[4] It's not ok, and it's not fair. Neither is menopause. We're even.[5]

Marriage doesn't fare so well when alcoholism is involved. If one spouse suffers from alcohol use disorder, it heightens the risk of divorce by 20 percent, and the divorce is more likely if the wife is the abusive drinker. Well, gee. I could have told the researchers this. Drinking first took my marriage and doused it with numb. Then, a few drinks in, it would heighten everything—good feelings and bad. There's only so much of that back-and-forth drama that can happen before something gives.

On the day that I finally decided to stop drinking, after a horrendous couple of weeks of off-the-charts binging, I still stubbornly held onto this thought: *I can do this myself. I don't need help.* Alcoholism constantly messes with you, and because up until then I had been either drunk, getting drunk, hungover, or sleeping, my ability to think clearly was impaired. I had tried to do this on my own before. I had tried to cut down. I had tried to drink only on the weekends, or only after five o'clock, or only when out for dinner. I failed all these tests. I failed the biggest test of all: being honest with myself.

Actually, what happened was, I called my husband and begged him to come home, and then hung up on him. And then I sat in the backyard and waited for him, and when he finally arrived and walked up the back sidewalk to me, I looked up blearily and said, "I need help. I have got to stop drinking and I can't." And Brian, to his credit, said nothing and just looked at me with very kind and very tired eyes.

And then I said, "But I am NOT going to meetings."

I never said I was perfect. Progress, not perfection, right?

I did get help. I did go to meetings. I had to. I had lobbed the "I'm too busy/ I have kids/ I don't know where the meetings are located/ I'm not into sharing" litany of excuses at my alcoholism long enough to know they were deadly, and they, along with the boxed wine, had to go. If I tried to do this on my own, something in me knew that I'd be worse the next time around. I wasn't sure I had a next time in me anymore.

And not once did Brian ever make me feel small. Not once did he use my alcoholism as a weapon. Not once. I'm proud of him for that. It would have been so easy.

But my recovery, as tough as it was on our relationship, didn't make things smaller for us. Our marriage now, versus those early years in recovery, is expansive. Recovery widened the horizon. Our relationship sees forward movement every day. Even on the worst days when I hate him and he hates me and we yell at each other and he's a slob and I'm a nag. It's still a forward movement because half of this marriage has an alcoholic in recovery in it. We are far from perfect, but the alcoholic half still goes to bed sober every day.

I had to stop looking for the payoff. I looked at so many things in my life with a "what's that gonna do for me?" mindset, and recovery cracked that open. I started to deal with life honestly, without any expectation of a return, just as a matter of being. And I look at my spouse, the number one relationship in my life, and I realize this: When I married this guy, I had so many expectations of a positive return on investment. He was going to make me happier.

Instead, what I learned was that he didn't have a whole lot to do with my happiness because it comes from me, and all that other annoying stuff you learn in recovery.

But there is one fun caveat: the Bacon Rule. If Brian is frying bacon for his ridiculously large Saturday breakfast that he makes, and even after asking me if I wanted a fried egg sandwich dripping with grease and cheese, and I say "no" because I like my arteries, I will STILL take at least two slices of his bacon. Even after I told him I wouldn't. Even after he asked me twice if I was sure. Because that is the Bacon Rule, and you don't mess with it. It's kind of the law.

I just love him. We are together. It's a total miracle how we found each other and that somehow we seem to balance each other pretty well on most days. He doesn't fix me. It's not bliss. That's the pay grade, and it's enough. In fact, it's riches.

Marriage: The Pros and Cons

Cons

Brian likes to use a tool in 2019 and then put it down where he used it, but up high, because he doesn't want it to get lost, and then forget that it was ever there. The rest of us in the house are short, so now the tool has left the chat. And so then, when he needs that tool five years later, he says things like, "Have you seen my side-radial gyrowrench? I could swear I put it right here. Did you move it?" But because you've been married for sixteen long years, you don't say this:

I have no idea what a side-radial gyrowrench even is and you never put your sh*t away, and I hate these questions because you KNOW I'm trying to work on myself and my issues with codependency (that's the next chapter), but STILL I'm gonna get up from whatever I'm doing and try to look, all the while muttering under my breath about you being tools-challenged, and no that's not code for something. And then, after about ten minutes of tension, you'll say, "Well! It's gone. Someone moved it! OH WELL IT DOESN'T MATTER I'LL JUST GO AND BUY ANOTHER ONE. IT'S ONLY MONEY" and stomp about, to which I kind of sigh and think, "I totally didn't see that comment coming" but I did. I did see it coming. This is the same conversation we've had about tools in this house for sixteen long years. Will it change? Never. What if I spend three thousand hours organizing and putting them all back in the really expensive tool containers we have? Still no. Acceptance is key.

Also, I have realized that for the rest of my life, I will be asked, "The yard looks good, doesn't it?"

Pros

A study found that couples who kiss goodbye each morning are less likely to get into car accidents. Vehicular safety has always been very important to Brian. He kisses me every morning without fail. Even if he is late. Even if we're in a fight. Even if I'm fast asleep and am snoring open-mouthed with fish breath. Without fail, he kisses me goodbye, doing his part to keep the roads hazard-free.

Notes

1 See what I did there?

2 Did you know that marriages actually fare better when there are pets involved? It's science. I have used this argument for the past year, lobbying for another cat. Brian says two cats and two dogs are enough, and now I'm getting irritated with him as I write this. This whole chapter has been a roller coaster of feelings about Brian, but he gave me permission to write it, so it's ok.

3   Actually this goes for all relationships. We alcoholics don't get to corner the market on acceptance.

4   We also came up with a code word for when Brian tried to mansplain things to me. I told him that if we don't have a code word, the next step would be yelling, so he agreed. He suggested "football." I suggested "asshole."

5   That is not a nice thing to say, Dana. That's just awful. How could you say such a thing for all these women who are also menopausal to read and deep down agree with?

Bibliography

1   **Winston Churchill's figurative "black dog" of depression:**
Daniels, Anthony M., and J Allister Vale (2018). Did Sir Winston Churchill Suffer from the "Black Dog"?. *Journal of the Royal Society of Medicine* 111 (11): 394–406. https://doi.org/10.1177/0141076818808428.

2   **Did you know that marriages actually fare better when there are pets involved?:**
Baker, Lois (1998, March 12). Pet-Owning Couples Are Closer, Interact More than Pet-Less Couples, UB Study Shows. https://www.buffalo.edu/news/releases/1998/03/3479.html.

3   **If one spouse suffers from alcohol use disorder, it heightens the risk of divorce by 20%:**
Lindner, Jannik (2023, December 16). Must-Know Alcohol and Divorce Statistics [Current Data]. *Gitnux*. https://tinyurl.com/4c6bjtce.

4   **A study found that couples who kiss goodbye each morning:**
Jain, Dr. Manoj (2014, December 13). A Kiss Is Not Just a Kiss: Biology vs. Psychology. *The Tennessean*. https://tinyurl.com/2bk59y8p.

8

The League of Good Women

A note from Dana: This chapter features some heavy discussion of my experience with depression and suicidal ideation. I won't feel bad if you want to jump to the next chapter if this isn't something you want to delve into at the moment.

My friend Jess and I are sitting on my front steps, and she hands me a coffee. Yesterday I texted her that I was struggling. The dogs of depression had come sniffing around my door again. And now, we are sitting and staring at my bedraggled lawn and I say,

"I feel tired and fat and old."

She says nothing, just leans in a bit. Her shoulder and arm are now firm along my side.

And then I say,

"And I don't want to talk about it."

More shoulder. No talk.

"Because I'm always talking about it. It gets annoying. Dana. With all her problems."

Jess shifts and turns to me. Her eyes are questions. I look down.

"I'm always bothering people with my problems."

Jess speaks. "Dana. Who told you that?"

I paused. "I think I did."

In my twenties, I wanted romantic love. I was very focused on this, like Ahab with his whale. It did not end well for Ahab, as those of us English majors know, but vigilant scanning of the horizon had served me well for many years, so the hunt began. Friends were in my life, but in a solid second-place slot. In my thirties, when loneliness and bitter heartache set in, friends comforted me and kept me close, but I didn't notice much. I was still wrapped tight in my sadness. Life was nothing if there was no love. My friends, again, placed a solid second. I had no idea how much I needed them. Still, they were relentless in their loyalty.[1] To this day, I am not sure why.

In my thirties, marriage and children came. This life came prepackaged with a new variety of friends: Moms. And just like that, I now belonged to a group of women with cute diaper bags and also with bags under our eyes. Oh, we were so tired. We couldn't get our babies to sleep. Does anyone have a good pediatrician to recommend? Ours doesn't seem to like children, to be honest. Did you try sleep training? No? Oh! You wear your baby? How? Show me. I need that wrap. I love that diaper bag. Where'd you get it? And your nails!? They're adorable! Oh, you sell them? And a pink drink? I'll buy!

Playdates started. In the early days, these were more for us than the babies. I attended. It was necessary, I knew, to make Mom friends because they are the only ones who will consistently hang out with me now. Single people will eventually drop me because children are sort of untranslatable to people who knew me before. But as both my sons made it into kindergarten, I realized: I didn't have to come along on these playdates anymore, and I sort of rejoiced. My social calendar had never involved so much social time, except in my college days, and even then, I preferred to work alone.

Moms, it's not you, it's me.

I'm the problem. It's me. Playdates and Lularoe and gossip about handsome pediatricians are wonderful. There were many times after a mom gathering when I would pack up my two toddlers into the car with the bags and snacks and a shoe because Henry wanted to wear just one, and sometimes an extra sippy cup that wasn't ours, and I would drive home and be kind of sad about myself. I had a good time with these Moms. We were comfortable, and I could show up in pajamas, and we could talk about it all: spouses, weariness, all of it.

But as we would all head home, I would be bothered because I was not bothered. I wanted to be alone. I didn't want to stay all day and talk and talk. I think I kind of figured that real friendship would mean that I would want that, but I didn't. Something in me was broken. I wasn't like the other moms.

Also, I was still a little hungover, and I needed to go home and have a lie down. I'd put on a Little Einsteins DVD, get the boys some lunch, and there would be quiet. I didn't *need* these mom friends. I had five best friends, none of whom lived in town, but I figured I was good. Bethany, Merri, Katie, Meredith, and Christy: The Five Wise Women. Five is a nice, solid number. That's all I needed, and anything extra was a nice surplus, like a backup pair of sunnies in case you misplace your Ray-Bans.

Let me tell you about my initial League of Good Women. Bethany has been with me since college. We met in the bathroom on the first night of our freshman year. She is defined by her kindness and her strong sense of justice. Amid the codependent mess that was my twenties, she hung in. Every once in a while, she would gently prod at me, at my drinking, at my twisty relationships. I never listened, but she loved me anyway. Merri and I had been best friends since working at Borders Bookstore in my twenties. She is an artist. I am looking at her painting on my wall as I write this, a large, exuberant floral work. It is celebratory and also calming, just as she is. Lately we had a talk about my perceived neediness and she said, "Well. That's bullshit. You have such LOVE in you, Dana!" She tends to speak in grand statements like that, like a walking billboard, and I need those capital letters in my life. Katie and Meredith, I met in my thirties. Katie is beautiful and fierce and funny. Meredith is beautiful and quiet and calm. They kept me sane during the codependent chaos of my thirties. I met Christy because her husband was Brian's friend. We were soulmates via our husbands. Brian and Karl are friends, yes, but Christy and I are FRIENDS.

All of these women are miracles in my life. All of these women hung on. They are tenacious, darling, and smart. But I moved away and saw them less and less, and they left a hole. One that I filled, I now realize, with my new best friend: alcohol.

So, what happened was, I got sober. I didn't get sober to mend friendships, or fix my marriage, or become a better mom. Honestly, in the early days, if someone asked me why I got sober, I'm not sure I would be able to give a reason. This was a lesson in humility. The good thing about humility is that it's abrasive. It scoured out my soul, and then whole rooms of me stood empty in an echoey way, like a house waiting, ready for occupants. That's when I started to understand my Mom friends better because I was dealing with reality now. Reality can be hard. I needed women in my life. I needed friends.

At this point in the story, it would be fitting if all the Moms answered back, "No way, Dana. You're too anti-social and weird. You kind of suck," and I was left with no one but Brian. But they didn't. And my Wise Women became eight, adding Kate, Amy, and Alissa. And then, because Alissa knows everyone, I now have the Twelve Mompostles. And now I promise I will stop with the biblical references.

And so, when Covid hit, and then menopause followed, I fell apart. Studies are just now discovering how the uncertainty of the pandemic really did a number on our brains. During lockdown and beyond, uncertainty caused us to revert back to fight or flight, but we also had to be normal-ish about it. Prolonged unpredictability saps motivation and focus. It whittles away at self-control, which would explain my fifteen-pound weight gain during the pandemic, and it made me unable to maneuver between different stages of the day: writing, helping a son with his endless math homework, and figuring out dinner. All of these things seemed more difficult, like suddenly normal, everyday life-ing had been turned up to impossible. But I didn't know that. I just slogged through, with a brain that was ratcheted up to "Everything is So Much Harder, but I Don't Know Why, and I Should Just Be Grateful We're Ok."

But these women, tenacious and a little bit sharky, kept circling. We texted. We congratulated each other on small wins ("Mike and I are actually going out. Woot" and we would respond with all the heart emojis. We asked for prayer (praying hands emojis). We wished happy birthdays (cake emojis).

We marked the little moments in our lives with each other (100 percent emojis). We loved and we emojied our way through all of it. We still do.

At one point, Alissa stalked me with a cup of coffee, walking around the back of my house and braving my two dogs so she could hunt me down. I spotted her hair first, bobbing by the fence line as I was hanging out some blankets to dry in the sun. She laughed as she approached, followed by her usual "How's it goin?" and "I found you!" Of all my friends, Alissa is the most extroverted in the bunch. She attends all the sports, even when her girls are not competing.

She does it just for fun. She works snack bars and heads fundraisers, and she is friends with every single person in our town. Probably the next town over, too. She stands with folks and drinks coffee, talks and smiles, and says things like, "How's Cooper? Did he get his cast off yet?" I can't understand how she not only knows everyone, but also their kids. She always has coffee and water, and probably a granola bar. She'll give you all three. She can find you a notary public; she'll tell you strawberries are on sale at Sam's Club, and she'll take candid shots of your kids because she's at their games and you're not, and text them to you.

Once, after a particularly stressful couple of weeks of impending deadlines, I wished I could head away on my own for a writer's retreat. She said, "I could never do that. I just like to spend time with my girls too much," and she actually means this. It sounds like it's mom-shamey, but she's incapable of that nonsense. Alissa is just really, really nice.

Alissa is in charge of us. She texts out about every six weeks or so and says, "Wanna meet for coffee?" Our schedules demand that 6 a.m. is the only time that works for us all, so we gather on Allison's rustic back porch in the darkness of early morning, drink lots of coffee, and watch the sunrise.

This group of moms? They changed my brain. In the face of uncertainty and the prolonged dreariness of Covid and beyond, their support showed me that optimism could be learned.

"Realistic optimism" is just what it sounds like. It's optimism, but it's smart about it. It has a backup plan. It's the Mom who shows up to all the sports events and gives hugs and a smile when your team loses by thirty-one points. Realistic optimists see all the possibilities that might play out, and she packs snacks and shows up early. Realistic optimism asks, "Yes, but what did you learn?" and not just at the end of that horrible basketball game, but also to this group of friends, right now, on Allison's back porch.

Actually, none of my friends ever says it that way. Nobody should ever look at someone who is struggling and say, "Well, but what did you *learn* after you lost your temper with your son because he lost HIS temper earlier, and then you felt like a total slug of a mom when you finally realized the irony? Hmmmm? But, what did you *learn*?"

Instead, this is what they said:

Allison: Been there. It's hard.

Jaime: Aw Dana. You need to be more gentle with yourself. Been there.

Jennifer: Yep. Me too.

Jess: Me too.

Laura: Me too.

Alissa: Me too. Just this morning, actually.

All of us eye Alissa with suspicion because we can't grasp that she yells at her kids. As I said, she's just so nice.

Alissa: What? I did! They really push your buttons sometimes! Here, I brought banana muffins. Try them.

All of this is a balancing act. We all air the pain and challenges of parenting on that back porch before sunrise. I don't feel placated. I don't feel misunderstood. If anything, I feel like the complexity of child-rearing is simplified with the ease of the "me too." Friendship trains my brain to regulate emotions. It's practiced and realistic optimism at its finest. One of us shares a failure or a fear, and the group gathers around and moves the fear gently from hand to hand, holding the moment. Lifting the moment. It's practical and it's real, and the brain responds very nicely by bulking up to do it more. Optimism actually increases the mass of the area of the brain that wards off anxiety. In other words, I meet up with these women, I share and listen and get a good dose of hope, and my brain stretches and smiles.

Practical help is the essence of realistic optimism. One early morning, after we shared about our kids and husbands and the best stuff we were reading, I mentioned that I was stressed about a website thing. "It's nothing, guys," I said apologetically, even though it had been bugging me for weeks. "I'm sure I'll figure it out." There was a beat. And then it began:

Within about five minutes, I had realistic advice, one phone number, two connections, a starting point, and hope. This plan worked, by the way, and my website is up and running today because of that 6 a.m. session. These women? They are the CEO's of living. I do what they say.

When I was in the last month of pregnancy with Charlie, I had severe back and leg problems that made walking difficult. I used to roll around on my desk chair while I taught middle school, feeling like a rollie walrus, scooting around to my students as we tried to learn about Edgar Allan Poe. I was exhausted. I was also extremely bothered by my increasingly messy house. The feeling that a baby was coming into a habitat of grime was not sitting well with me. And that's when my sister, Sherry, a card-carrying member of the League of Good Women, drove five hours with a car full of cleaning supplies and Italian food. For about three days, Shery cleaned my house from top to bottom. She also had vats of red sauce and sausage and pasta, and so much garlic bread that it nearly made me tearful. I lumbered around with my ice pack, waddling to the bathroom every ten minutes and then falling back into bed, asleep. My stomach would rumble, and she'd bring me more garlic bread. At one point, she came into the bedroom, out of breath, and said, "The floor. In the bathroom. Is clean." She shook her head with a traumatized look in her eyes. Up to that point, I had a messy, kind of clean house. But now, it had been Sherry-cleaned. My house would never be the same.

I was never the same. I never forgot that Sherry did that for me. Ever. I mean, I think if she had had more time, she would have organized our attic for us or perhaps built a back deck. She would have fixed everything.

She offered practical help, and she gave me exactly what I longed for at the time: a clean place from which to start.

That's what friendship does. It gives us a clean place from which to start.

My other sister, Jenni, and her brand of help in my life are not practical at all. What Jenni does is send me texts and snaps constantly telling me how freaking amazing I am. Here's an example:

Me: Sends video of a mom cat hugging her kitten.

Jen: Hilarious! Just like you! You're the best! You're the funniest, darling sis! Also, you're the best mom ever! And, just in general! Like, everything you do is the best! There is literally nothing in this world that you can do wrong! Like, nothing! I love you!

Being the recipient of this firestorm of wonderfulness could make a person jaded. I could receive all this and think, "Sure. I bet that's what she says to all the girls," and the thing is, Jen does. She is like this with everyone, and also? She *fricking means* it. She's been this way her whole life; always weirdly fond of me, always willing to head the cheerleading squad. Is it delusional? Probably. Do I massively benefit? Yes. Everyone should have a Jen in their life, too. We all need someone who is so blatantly nutty in the encouragement department.

Well, unless you're an oligarch. Kim Jong Un doesn't need a Jen, but maybe if he'd had one in his past, North Korea wouldn't be so horrible today.

Oh, and don't get me started on my mom. She is sweet and small and offers really good advice in long letters written in tiny script. But also? Don't cross her. She does not suffer fools, and she will cut you.

These women. They are necessary. They don't take us around. They don't have *time* for that. They take us straight through.

Back when I was starting on all my medical appointments for the menopausal symptoms, I started noticing something else that was becoming a struggle—an incessant buzzing sound in my ears. I can't really pinpoint when this started, but one night as I was lying on the couch watching a movie, I noticed it. The movie was the quiet kind because I was blessedly alone, so I was watching something with dialogue and no explosions. And, amid the dialogue and long, thoughtful silences, I heard it. A buzzing, like a cicada, was stuck in my head. I sat up and yawned, pulling on an ear. That . . . noise. Had it always been there? Was this new? Was I imagining it?

I figured I was imagining it. It was probably allergies. I was probably just getting a headache.

The buzzing increased over the passage of two years. I felt crazy. I tried to explain to Brian, but "incessant buzzing" didn't cover it anymore. Now, I had a sports arena of cicadas in my head. My ears felt swollen, and the only thing that helped was lying on an ice pack at night. I dreaded the quiet. I dreaded sleep again. I sometimes felt like I might go crazy, just absolutely nuts, from the persistent screeching.

I read up. I asked my doctor. I was told it was tinnitus, and I couldn't get help for it. There was no known cure. Melissa gave me a supplement but explained that it "might help, but it might not," and I took it for months. It didn't help.

Sometimes I cried. It felt a bit like torture.

But then, I felt dumb. It wasn't Covid. It wasn't cancer. I shouldn't be throwing words like "torture" around. Once again, I shrugged and sighed and told myself not to make a mountain out of a shrieking medical molehill.

But, I couldn't hear. I taught classes. Nearly every time a student responded to a question, I had to ask her to repeat it. Sometimes I would walk up close, lean in, and even place a hand behind my ear. By the way, this kind of thing?

It freaks a college student out. My relationship with my students had become geriatric now, and I started to nod a lot when they commented, not ever completely sure what I was nodding to. I stopped asking so many questions. I felt far away.

My relationship with my husband now consisted of us yelling "What?!" at each other about ninety percent of the time. This was a marked rise from the normal thirty percent of "What?!"-ing over the years. I was irritated with him more. I felt far away.

And, my boys. The poor darlings. They kept saying things like "yeet" and "bussin,"[2] and I did think I was going crazy. I needed to learn a new language, and I couldn't hear it. I felt very, very far away.

Sometimes it was just easier to stay quiet, to not ask any questions. I felt far away, so I ended up going over there, far away, and I sat down and got quiet.

Finally, my friend Suzanna spoke up (in a loud and clear voice). She said this: DANA. EVERYTHING I SAY TO YOU I HAVE TO SAY TWICE. MAYBE YOU HAVE A HEARING PROBLEM? YOU SHOULD GO TO THE DOCTOR.

But it's . . . just tinnitus. It's not hearing *loss*. It's just the screeching thing. Besides, I was getting through the choke-sleeping, and depression, and working through 8 a.m. doom feelings. I have enough going on.

And maybe. Just perhaps. I was afraid.

This weird hearing thing was starting to feel bigger than just a hearing thing. I had been ignoring it for over a year, so I was well-practiced at avoidance. And I was very afraid that trying to deal with it, making more appointments, trying to get to the bottom of something that I was being told was just in my head, I feared **that**. I was afraid of being afraid again, which is the essence of anxiety.

Ok, as long as we're being honest, I also felt old.

The Good Women gathered around. They suggested an audiologist. They asked me to get pink hearing aids because those would match my outfits. One of them told me she'd accompany me to the appointment. They joked with me about feeling old because we joke about stuff like that, and we were in this together, remember? Remember, Dana? We've been *over* this. You seem to forget it all the time, but you're not alone. You feel far away, but it's time to go through it again, to come closer. And I listened.

Even though I couldn't hear a damn thing.

I went to the audiologist. Emily is also a Good Woman, but she is in her twenties, so she's Junior League. She has good wavy hair, and each time I went to see her, I wanted to ask her about what products she used. After my initial hearing tests, she ushered me out of the soundproofed room and settled me back in her office. Then, she asked me, "Were you like a roadie for a band or something?" I laughed and shook my head. "Did you go to a lot of concerts?"

The last concert I attended was Earth, Wind and Fire's revival tour, where everybody was my age, so nobody could figure out how to turn on their phone flashlight for the slow ballad. Other than that, I didn't go to concerts. They never started on time, and you had to stand a lot. She shook her head. "Well, you have pronounced hearing loss. That, paired with the tinnitus . . . I'm surprised you didn't come in sooner."

I said, "Well. I kept thinking it was all in my head." She blinked at me and said, rather gently,

"Well, yes. It is. Your ears are right up there, in your," and she gestured around her perfect hair—"head." Well played, Emily.

She fitted me with a trial pair of hearing aids. And she leaned back and said, "How's that sound?" I didn't respond. I just sat there doing this dramatic "mouth dropping open" thing. After a minute, I said, "This is what it should sound like?" She smiled and nodded. The buzzing was muted. My ears felt lighter, not heavy. If this is possible, it felt like two little doors had been opened in them. Sound was there. I think it was all a bit much because my eyes filled with tears.

She smiled and said, "It's a bit much, right? It's ok."

"No. Yes. I don't know."

Hearing is so underrated.

I left the appointment with hearing aids on. I was now a hearing aid wearer. And I didn't care, not one bit. I had no idea what I had been missing. As Emily led me to the exit, I turned to her and said, "Can I give you a hug?" and she answered, "Of course, you can give me a hug." And as she did so, she said, "This is my favorite part of the job. People come in, and people leave, totally different."

I walked out to my car, and I swore I could hear someone dropping a piece of paper down the block. In the next town, a bird chirped. I felt like Spiderwoman.

All my girlfriends asked to see the hearing aids. They were "champagne toned,"³ not pink, and everyone said they barely noticed them. "But, you can HEAR! That's a miracle!" said Jess. "Who cares if you can see them!" I nodded. I was wearing miracles.

The next thing I am going to say is so very cheesy, it might not make it into the final edits. I imagine my editor will read what's next, slap her hands down on the table with, "Well, that's it! I have reached cheese capacity," and cross it all out. I don't know. But it's true. It's really true:

I got the hearing aids. And then, I made a promise to listen more. Because that's what friendship is. It's listening. Really listening.

And finally, I have Kayla.

When the depression got really bad, I didn't want to seek help. That's depression's thing. It's not a visible malady, like my arm just fell off, so it gets ignored. But because I know how to do this agonizing thing called Taking Care of Myself, I google psychiatrists in my area. It is overwhelming. I find one close by. It probably won't work—the psychiatrist will be booked until next year, or insurance will say no, or she'll be three hours away. I sigh. I keep going. I make a call. I don't believe, but I act like I do.⁴

I had an appointment set up with this woman, Kayla, within the week. I spent the days pushing my thoughts around, staring at ceilings in the morning, and contemplating canceling. Kayla will probably be awful. She'll be a wrong fit, and there will be a whole afternoon wasted, and I am just so tired. Wouldn't a nap be a better idea?

This woman, Kayla? She saved my life.

Kayla and I met on a Thursday morning, and I prepared myself for the familiar onslaught of questions. This is what you do at the first appointment. You answer a bunch of questions that you've answered a million times before, and you try to be specific even though your memory can't really hold onto anything specific anymore. Kayla asked me about my family, my work, and my hobbies. She asked about all my medications, and of course, I forgot about the dosage, but I remembered that I kept all that on my phone now. Then, I forgot where. I started fiddling around on my phone, and she probably typed "Has memory of fruit fly" into her records at that point, but then she said it was no big deal. She'd get this information from my doctor.[5] All the while, she stared at her computer screen and tapped away while asking me questions. I sat in my chair, quietly waiting, wondering briefly how many forms about Dana were out there, swirling around from doctor to doctor, with things like "not sleeping well" and "on a scale of one to ten, feels despair at nine" and "works well with others" on them.

I sighed. Kayla stopped typing, folded her hands in front of her, and looked at me. She said, "Tell me why you're here," and I shrugged like a sullen teenager. I wanted to say, "I'm not really sure anymore," but instead I explained the visits to my doctor about the sleep-choking thing and the menopause diagnosis.

"Well, and," I took a breath. "Um, alongside that . . . I'm kind of having a hard time."

She nodded. "Having a hard time. Can you explain?"

I shifted. "You know . . . just tired, but that's probably because of the lack of sleep." She nodded again. "And, I guess, you know. I am feeling depressed. But I know I get this way," I waved my hand around my head, "sometimes."

Then Kayla asked me something I don't remember any counselor ever saying to me. "What does it feel like? Like, in your body, when you 'get this way'?"

I looked down. "It feels like . . . weight. My heart aches—it hurts, I mean. It feels like it can't pump properly. And everything I do or think or touch, it feels coated with dread."

She took a breath. Then said, "Like, you have to brush your teeth but—"

"But I can't. It's dread. It's dead weight."

"And right now, as you're sitting here, is there that weight?"

I didn't realize I was crying now. Big hot tears silently dripping. I nod.

"Ok, on a scale of one to ten, ten being the worst—"

"Ten." I say it so softly. I don't look at her. "Ten."

In the softest, gentlest voice, she said: "Do you want to die, Dana?"

I don't expect that. I look up. I try to rally. "No. No, I don't." But then I take a breath and try to think of a way to explain it. "I don't want to die . . . I just don't want to be here anymore." I'm back to looking at my hands, tightly clasped in my lap, and the wedding ring on my finger. I don't want to be here. Where did that come from? Really? That's dramatic, Dana. You're just being dramatic.

In the smallest voice ever, I try again. "I just want to be left alone."

There was a silence. And then she said, "Well. I'm not going to allow that."

I was still tired, but with her help, we got to work.

Honesty meant that we discussed hospitalization. We talked about suicidal ideation, and I was making plans to carry this out, along with all those awful, horrible, awkward things that had to be talked about. I was honest about it. No, I didn't have a plan in place for killing myself. Yes, at least once or twice a day, I was having thoughts that were along the lines of "not wanting to be here." She patiently asked me, prodded me, and made me tell the truth. And as I sat there and kept trying to piece it together, I also started to realize something. I think I could really trust this woman.

We decided together that hospitalization wasn't the plan at this time, but it would be if these thoughts persisted. She used the words "clinical depression" and suggested an immediate change in my meds, telling me about a different antidepressant that had better results with menopausal women. "Sometimes when you've been taking the same prescription for a really long time, your brain needs a change-up. You've been taking the same med for nearly twenty years, Dana," she said, and remarkably, this didn't make me feel impatient or jaded about trying something new. It made sense.

She gave me her cell phone number. We made a plan for the next appointment. There was also a prescription for sleeping that wasn't addictive and wouldn't make me buy movie soundtracks in the middle of the night. She explained the research. I trusted her. I trusted what she was telling me. It was a risk, yes, because she could be completely wrong, but my gut was telling me that Kayla wasn't wrong.

Kayla wasn't wrong. With two new prescriptions and a better grip on a plan for my mental health, I started feeling better within three weeks. I slept through the night more often. I didn't fear bedtime. I didn't fear my feelings so much, either, because I had Kayla.

Everybody needs a Kayla. She listened and advocated and told me after about three visits, "You look different today. The first time I met you, you were . . . not you." She smiles at me. "**Now** you're here." She smiled at that, and I smiled back. I had forgotten how to see myself anymore, and Kayla was showing me how.

The official diagnosis is clinical depression, paired with bouts of mania that last about two to three days every couple of months. Bipolar disorder was a possibility, but she wanted to wait on that. I told her I kind of loved the mania stuff. "It's when I can get stuff done."

She smirked. "Yes . . . but that's not the best way to do it, huh?" I nodded and rolled my eyes. Yes, Kayla. I know. Geez.

These relationships with these women? It gives me hope. And I really need that right now. They lead me back to self-efficacy when I forget the way. Solidarity makes us healthier. Literally. Having friends reduces our risk of chronic illness. People with friends live longer. Friend-laden brains *thrive*. And, I'm biased, but women's friendships? We are a totally special thing. We are in a league of our own.

In one of my favorite psychological studies, participants guessed that the hill they were walking up was less steep if they could take a friend with them on the journey. Friends help us up, and then they help us through. They squash hills. That's what the League of Good Women does. They are superheroes, after all.

So what if . . . Mom friends took over the world?

Here are the texts.

Mom group subs in during World Leaders' Summit:

Mom 1: Ok, so we are here to try and solve a whole bunch of problems.

Mom 2: I made a text group for all of us.

Mom 3: Banana muffins if you're feeling hangry. The people in these meetings always look hangry.

Mom 4: Is there fresh coffee? I feel like we need some coffee. And the nice creamer.

Mom 3: Yep! I brought three different kinds of creamer. It's always good to have a variety.

Mom 1: So, here's problem #1. Mom 5 made a nice graphic for us.

Mom 2: That is so fab! I am awful at technology. I love it!

Mom 1: It's seriously the best graphic ever.

Mom 5: Aw, thanks, guys. I used to do this back when I was working. Now I just stay at home—

Mom 1: Do not EVEN say you just stay at home! World's toughest job! You know it!

All Moms: YES

Mom 6: Uh, guys? I have a thought. (Pulls out whiteboard with several colored markers.) Why don't we just move this stuff around here and put this stuff over there? It's just like our family calendar at home.

Mom 1: That is awesome! I love it!

Mom 2: I agree! And all we need to do then is help that one group apologize to the other group. We can walk them through it, surely? Maybe? Like, I'm not sure if anyone has a better idea . . .

Mom 1: I think you both fixed it. Yep. Great collab! Done and dusted.

Mom 7: OMG, I am so sorry. Cooper had a doctor's appointment.

Mom 3: No worries! We are so glad you're here! Have a muffin?

Mom 7: Holy cow, these are so good. I swear; one piece of it could solve all the world's problems. Recipe, please!

Mom 3: Yea! I'll put it in the text group.

Mom 4: Let's get a pic before we leave, ok?

Mom 3: And take a muffin before you go!

Notes

1   Thank you.

2   These terms will be uncool at printing. While I worked on this chapter, I texted my son repeatedly while he was trying to be a good kid in school, asking him what kids were saying these days. I apologize, teachers, for texting my son at school. It was just really important that I understand what in the actual hell skrt skrt means.

3   Hit up with alcohol-flavored hearing aids. Alcoholic irony for the win.

4   There's a verse in the bible that says something like, "Lord, I believe. Help me in my unbelief." and that's what people in recovery do. We act as if we believe and put one foot in front of the other. Even when it's hard. Especially when it's hard.

5   HUGE GREEN FLAG. Communicating with my other medical providers? Mind blown.

Bibliography

1. **Studies are just now discovering how the uncertainty of the pandemic really did a number on our brains:**
Grant, Heidi, and Tal Goldhamer (2021, September 22). Our Brains Were Not Built for This Much Uncertainty. *Harvard Business Review*. https://hbr.org/2021/09/our-brains-were-not-built-for-this-much-uncertainty.

2. **'Realistic optimism' is just what it sounds like:**
Dawson, Chris, and David de Meza (2020, July 7). Why Realism Is the Key to Wellbeing – New Research. *The Conversation*. https://tinyurl.com/4d6jhppn.

3. **Friendship trains my brain to regulate emotions:**
Newman, Kira (2021, February 8). How Friends Help You Regulate Your Emotions. *Greater Good*. https://greatergood.berkeley.edu/article/item/how_friends_help_you_regulate_your_emotions.

4. **Optimism actually increases the mass of the area of the brain that wards off anxiety:**
Bergland, Christopher (September 23, 2015). Optimism and Anxiety Change the Structure of Your Brain. *Psychology Today*. https://www.psychologytoday.com/us/blog/the-athletes-way/201509/optimism- and-anxiety-change-the-structure-your-brain.

5. **They lead us back to self-efficacy when we forget the way:**
Guerrero, Mayra, Casey Longan, Camilla Cummings, Jessica Kassanits, Angela Reilly, Ed Stevens, and Leonard A. Jason (2022). Women's Friendships: A Basis for Individual-Level Resources and Their Connection to Power and Optimism. *The Humanistic Psychologist* 50 (3): 360–75. https://doi.org/10.1037/hum0000295.

6. **Having friends reduces our risk for chronic illness:**
Rauchman, Brianna (2023, February 9). Social Health: Friends Are the Secret to a Healthy Brain. *Pacific Neuroscience Institute*. https://tinyurl.com/ycxe2ze8.

7. **. . . participants guessed that the hill they were walking up was less steep if they could take a friend with them on the journey:**
Schnall, Simone, Kent D. Harber, Jeanine K. Stefanucci, and Dennis R. Proffitt (2008). Social Support and the Perception of Geographical Slant. *Journal of Experimental Social Psychology* 44 (5): 1246–55. https://doi.org/10.1016/j.jesp.2008.04.011.

9

Veggie Rehab

My first experience of eating pizza with Brian involved a restaurant where everyone was very cheerful and Italian, even though they weren't Italian. Little green, red, and white flags were stuck everywhere. Candles in Chianti bottles dripped on the paper tablecloths. Lady and the Tramp were seated next to us. Every table had a bottle of house wine on it, and right away we filled our glasses, and I loved this place. Wine! Right here! No waiting! As I drank the stuff and slowly sank back into the red vinyl booth, I felt Italian too, in a Disney sort of way, all large colors and sounds.

We ordered pizza. When the waitress hoisted a huge steaming pan across the dining room toward our table, the pizza shouted at us. "Hey! I'm WALKIN' here!" The waitress had to dramatically shove all of our cutlery out of the way to accommodate its girth.

This pizza was not really a pizza. It was like a drawer of cheese. It was so crammed with all the things that were supposed to make it pizza that whenever you tried to cut into it, it sort of reanimated itself to its original size. It frightened me.

Ok, it was delicious. You can't go wrong when you order a drawer of cheese. I ate about 1/78 of the pizza, and we bundled the rest up into a takeout box that I cradled like a baby as we left.

We walked out into the cold night. It was quiet, and I breathed in the cool air. That restaurant had been sort of an immersive event, and I really needed to decompress. So, I looked at Brian and said, "Wanna go to a bar?"

Bars are not all that decompressive. But I am an alcoholic, did you know? If anyone back then offered, "Hey, you're tired and strung out, let's go someplace loud and inebriated to celebrate this!" I turned into a Pavlovian alcoholic.

We went to O'Malley's, ordered more alcohol, and at the end of the evening, I remember only one detail with assurance: We left our drawer of cheese behind. Since then, Brian and I have been leaving takeout containers behind about 75 percent of the time. It's our thing. We want something for them to remember us by.

Because I am an English teacher, that pizza became a symbol. Its layers and the weight of it, the never-ending strings of goo and delight, became my desire when it came to food. Somehow, I feared there would never be enough, so I wanted all of it. I wanted excess to the point of absurdity. If I could be so brazen as to add another metaphor to all these literary dives I'm taking: I was kind of the Imelda Marcos of food.

For example, I am now married to an appetizer man. When I was a kid, if we went out to a restaurant, there were rarely appetizers. Appetizers were too much. They would ruin our dinner. I think for a long time I never really even knew they existed.[1]

But when I married Brian, something wild happened when we would go out to eat. He would peruse the menu and then lean in and say, "Do you want any appetizers?" and I would say, "Oh no . . . that's . . . no. That's too much. They'll just ruin my dinner." And he'd say, "Really? You sure?" because every question he has ever asked me in our marriage has to be fact-checked.[2] And I would think, Hey. Maybe I do want some appetizers after all. I mean, I just basically found out they were a thing, so why not? Why not live a little?

And then we'd order appetizers, and I'd be in heaven. Appetizers are so *good*, y'all. They're fried and there's that great feeling of variety-nosh. With great attention, I would try a little bit of each. After that, I would eat four bites of my main course because I was full, only to package it all up and leave it on the table.

Brian is also a dessert person, and that about blew my head off. What is this sorcery? Italian wedding cake? Want to try it? Why sure! Brownie sundae when you're already half-sick from all the appetizers? Live a little! Bread pudding that comes in a cute little mini skillet and thunks down on the table with a delicious weight? Where have you been all my life?

Where, indeed.

There has been a lot of food fear in my life. The fear said, "You will never change," and I listened. I feared I would never have enough. I feared, I guess, that I would never be enough. I feared never feeling good in my skin, and never really loving a salad, like my Tiny Mom friends. We know those Tiny Moms, the ones we love and also hate a bit, because they coo, "Oh, I love a good salad," and mean it.

Over half of Americans report that they are stressed out. Stress levels have increased by nearly 78 percent since the pandemic, and those numbers still show upward movement. One million people in the United States call in sick every day due to stress. But stress is often labeled as an "I'll deal with this later" issue, so it's largely just tolerated. Nearly every doctor's visit I attended was paired with this fun question: Do you have a lot of stress in your life? To which I would chuckle. I mean, don't we all? And, really? How would you like me to unhook from my daily existence? Take the kids and the husband and the dogs and the elderly cat and the back gate that is broken and the lack of healthy snacks and strawberries that are full of pesticides and the election and that weird stomach pain I've been having, and just . . . boot them all? Really? How? How do you reduce stress when it just looks at you and nuttily refuses? It's Glen Close in *Fatal Attraction* with the wild hair and smeared eyeliner, warning, "I will not be IGNORED, Dana!" But you do ignore it, just like Michael Douglas did. This is not going to end well.

It's everywhere and all the time, and I don't see it anymore. Well, that's not true. I see stress. I nod at it as I jet by because I forgot to buy a birthday card for my friend. Stress and I? We cohabitate, I guess. Women do tend to be more aware of the strain in our lives, maybe because we talk about it more. My league of good women and I will share. We've got thirty-seven things on our to-do list for the day, and only about two of them have to do with our own lives. The rest is relational. There is no stopping for that.

And maybe, just perhaps, we wave the stress flag to normalize it and fit in. It's a mom thing.

Maybe, just maybe, it's a badge.

When the boys were toddlers, I remember my friend Amy asking if I was going to attend some get-together that evening. I was at her house for a playdate, and I looked at her and shook my head. "Oh no," I said. "That's against my rule. I only do One Thing a Day." She blinked at me. "I mean, I do this," and gestured at one kid who had taken off a sock and was chewing on it while the other batted him in the head with a tinker toy. "But it's my One Thing for today. Then we're heading home." She started laughing.

"Seriously? Only one thing a day? How can you manage that?" Introvert moms reading this might sigh a little. We don't. It's impossible. I wasn't able to keep my One Thing rule intact at all because I didn't have a grip on reality. Once my children were in school, they signed up for every known sport and music event available. They wanted to join it all, and I felt proud of them, but I also wilted a little inside. I bought all the picture packages and went to all the things, and my One Thing life faded away, like a sweet dream, along with my ability to drink non-alcoholically.

I think my One Thing rule originated from something I did as far back as my twenties, when I participated in my own sporting event called Do Nothing Day. About once a semester, I would call in sick, and I would lie in bed and read and eat Twizlers for the *entire day*. I would get up for water. That's about it. Maybe I'd watch my *Princess Bride* VHS or reruns of Family Ties. I never got out of my pajamas, and my dog Norman and I would medal in inertia.

I realize now that this was my version of a mental health day. And it was lovely, until about 5 p.m. But then, surrounded by *Delia's* catalogs and candy wrappers on my couch, a creeping dread would sink into me. The fear and stress about the next day would hit, along with a strong sense of shame. "You are so lazy," my brain would tell me. My feelings would respond with "Yes, and lazy people are awful. You are just awful," and so on. I would try to avoid the grumblings and dread in my head by adding a takeout meal from Chili's and a whole lot of wine.

I think Do Nothing Day sounds kind of dreamy today. I would appreciate you, Do Nothing Day. I wouldn't take you for granted. I would savor the moments, but just so you know, there would be no wine. Just a pile of good books and my front porch, and no shame. Maybe I'd take a nap around 3 p.m., and I would wake up when *my eyes opened by themselves*, not because someone is asking me where a charger cord is. I'm pretty sure there would be a cat in there, too.

Someday, Do Nothing Day, you and I are getting back together.

Research indicates that women respond to stress more emotionally than men. We feel stress, and portions of the brain that register anxiety and lower emotional resilience light up, and then whammo, food cues zap us. We have brains that say, "Feed me!" when we are upset. This is frustrating. Why can't my brain say, "Sign up for a marathon!" when I get overwhelmed? But, I can't anyhow because my kids have already entered one, and I have to go watch them.

By the way, I would also eat when I was happy, confused, or bored. I could go for months without ever feeling physical hunger. Feelings would slowly tick past me like that wheel on The Price is Right, and anywhere the arrow would stop would mean a snack. Back when I was drinking, it meant a snack plus wine. It's hard to walk away from a habit like that when it's all I've done for over twenty years. And stress is linked to addiction because, of course, it is. Why not make stress a little more stressful?

So, here's a scenario. I like to call this:

Dinner: A Tragedy in One Act

Henry is in the living room with his cello. He's supposed to be practicing for his upcoming concert, but instead, he's trying to figure out how to play Danger Zone from *Top Gun*. He just repeats it. Over. And over. I'm in the kitchen, where the dogs have moved into their one-on-one defense positions, waiting for me to carry something, preferably a casserole. Then they will stand directly in front of me, in hopes that a foul might mean crumbs. I am unable to take two steps in either direction for the duration of the play. My husband is late, and any attempts to contact him result in "Hi, you've reached Brian Bowman. Please leave a message—" in a much more cheerful voice than he should be using. I text WERE RU because I have left grammar behind. I'm attempting to make a healthy meal, but I get distracted by the dryer buzzing and both cats meowing from the top of the stairs, so the meal will be slightly singed. It had potential, but now it's just leathery, like a 1990s starlet.

I try to finish the potatoes, but the masher is in the dishwasher, and then I realize I need to empty the dishwasher, which reminds me we need soap, and there might be some in the basement, but I have to get shoes on to go down there because my basement is where crickets go to die. When I round the corner to get my shoes, I find out that Rey, the dog, has gacked all over the one area in the living room that has a rug on it. I can't remember where I put the rug cleaner; I think it's also in the basement, and I remember the shoes, but then I look at the fourteen pairs of shoes by the front door, and none of them are mine. This makes me go upstairs to get shoes, carrying a laundry basket, two library books, and some Flonase that has been sitting at the bottom of the stairs since 2015. I lay these down in our bedroom and then stare, wondering what brought me up here. And that's when I hear a cat gakking in solidarity with Rey, and I wonder if all our pets are dying and how horrible that would be, but also so much better for our carpets.

And that's when I feel it, a tiny "pa-ching!" in my brain. It was my last synapse that was holding on to sanity with its tiny stressed-out hands, and it just snapped.

Dinner congeals. The husband gets home late and says, "Well, something sure smells good!" which I take as idiocy, and I serve up a rage salad and leathery chicken. Nobody eats much, and I hate everyone except the pets, and even they are suspect at this point. But, they all might be dying, so then I feel guilty.

As a final act, Brian and I get into an argument about nasal spray. "They're all over the house!" I sigh. "It's like we're decorating with them. We have Flonase in at least five different places, and we need to collate them. They need to be in one spot!" This is just the type of argument a married couple has at an 8 p.m. dinner where tiredness and anger are slowly curdling. I realized later that I was the one who brought the Flonase upstairs and that this whole conversation had been a fight with myself. My grasp on control weakens further still.

I have had healthy food all day. I ate lentils for lunch because I know lentils are good for me, and I am trying to like them even though they taste like dirt. I had a salad and some fruit. Oatmeal. Yogurt. It's been a healthy eating day, and I am proud of myself. I eat the leathery chicken and I think, "Well, I am full. I am nicely full," and everything is fine. Stress had circled the wagons in preparation for warfare, but then things settled down, and I had a nice nutritional meal to end my day. Now, I'm going to have a cup of hot tea and head to bed, and it's good. I mean, tonight was just the same as every other night, really. And I brush my teeth and moisturize, and I don't forget to floss, and I open my book.

And then I get up and put on a robe and go downstairs and eat everything in our kitchen that is made out of flour.

The End

Stress stays in my body and waits. When I finally take a breath and think, "Well, now I have passed it on by," stress interjects. "Well, *actually*, Dana? You're not *really* relaxed. Food has to happen now, even though that won't help you feel calm. But let's give it a go, anyway." Stress continues, stressplaining. "This is what you *do*, Dana. This is how you have trained yourself to understand 'relaxed.' Some people just do deep breaths or meditation, but you? You do Captain Crunch."

One morning, I changed my mind. I didn't change my mind about disordered eating or my lack of willpower or the binging. I changed my mind about my mind.

I was standing at the kitchen sink in the early morning, feeling tired and achy from too much sugar the night before. Sugar now had a direct physical effect on me, causing joint pain and shaky unease the next day, like a donut hangover. Gazing out my kitchen window, I thought, "You seriously need to get a grip on food." This is the same mental path I've been taking for over thirty years. I cling harder to this logic by adding the usual, "Let's make a plan. Let's write some lists. Let's google. Let's attack this with control and ideas." And, because my brain loves repetition, this was followed by a sigh of frustration. "But this won't work. I hope it works, but it probably won't because you will never change." And then, I would finally land on fear. "It's always going to be like this."

I took a breath. "I don't want to live this way," I said. My brain nodded and said, "Well, let's start with some lists and some ideas and try—"

"No," I said. "I mean. I don't care about this anymore. I guess. I can keep screwing up, but I don't want to attach all these feelings to it."

I probably didn't say that out loud. It was far too early for me to be so vulnerable over a kitchen sink, but something in my head changed. For ages and ages, it felt like I kept trying to change my mind about my eating when instead, I needed to change my mind about my *feelings* about eating.

This would be crazy. It wouldn't be possible. I might as well attempt walking on water. But I'd dealt with the surface tension of my eating habits for so long that I was ready to try. Each time a particularly bad incident would occur—a late-night binge, or a whole slew of days where I ate only junk food and carbs and started to feel sluggish and hopeless and stunned, I would try to do a deep dive into all the reasons why, all the ways I could fix it, and all the things I should *do*. I'd plunge into plans and worry that I couldn't solve it, and eventually, the struggle would become evident from any shoreline. I'd drown.

Oh, how I longed to just float along, barely touching the surface of my feelings, just staring at the sky. And that morning, with my kitchen sink and the possibility of another day, at the exact time when normally I would be getting out a saucepan to make some lentils and embarking on yet another program of reno-Dana, I let it go. I decided to float. Light things float. It wasn't my eating that was making me heavy; it was the shame.

This sounds like ignorance is bliss. Perhaps it is. But here's what happened next.

I decided to forgive myself, but badly.

My mom taught me long ago that if you don't like something, but you still have to suck it up and do it, you "act as if," you like it. This is a recovery thing. She learned it in Al-Anon. Dad knows about it, but he's never brought it up. I'm pretty sure Dad thinks "acting as if" is too namby-pamby and he doesn't "act" anything. He MAKES it so. My mom and I are not quite as tough as Jim, so we just fake a lot of our lives, and I'm ok with that. It does work, by the way. Is it non-genuine and inauthentic at first? Sure. Maybe. Does it seem a little like you're lying to yourself? Why, that's entirely possible! Does it weirdly work anyhow and eventually make you accept the very thing you originally were all pissy about? Yes! It's magical thinking in a way that works. I love magical thinking!

So, I decided to forgive myself, but very half-assedly. I just *acted* as if I did. "I forgive you, Dana, for all this food crud," I muttered. I was a little sullen about it. But, I acted *as if* I actually could forgive the years of messing up my brain when it came to eating. I acted as if I forgave myself for being a stupid alcoholic with all this stupid addiction crap that has plagued me for ages. I acted as if I cared about forgiving, even when I pretty much knew it would not work, and this was all utterly dumb. I acted as if I wasn't mad about it all and sick and tired and, yes, still ashamed, and I forgave and forgave and did what I would like to think of now as apologizing to myself really REALLY badly.

This is also known as Shitty Forgiveness: Level One.

But, I did it.

And then I decided to go for Shallow Forgiveness: Level Two by deciding that my feelings could hang out in Level One. They could just stay the hell over there. Level Two would be as feelings-free as humanly possible. I would be a completely shallow ingrate with my forgiveness, no thinking allowed. I would ignore feelings and just mechanically do the forgiving and then go do something else, even eat four donuts if I wanted to, and *not think about it*. If this level were a movie, it would be *Sharknado*. If it were a song, it would be Baby Shark. For once, I would allow my feelings to slide on by, blips of "Huh, I'm feeling that. La la la la la!" and repeat.

Does any of this sound weird? Exhaustion will do that to you. I decided to take on forgiveness with the emotional depth of Beavis and Butthead and it was a total betrayal of everything I believe in, but I didn't freaking care anymore.

Incidentally, "fake it till you make it" has been scientifically proven to work. A study on botox injectors who were unable to frown post-injection reported that they felt happier after the procedures. Acting as IF you are happy, just because frowning has been incapacitated by a big ol' needle stimulates the amygdala, the emotion center of the brain. The amygdala is part of what some refer to as "lizard brain," where thinking doesn't hunker down. The amygdala reacts and positions itself as the bro in the back row who blurts out stuff. So, my decision not to think about forgiveness should be backed solidly by the non-thinking center of my brain, which kind of sounds like some presidential campaign strategies.

But, remember, I don't really care about any of this sciencey stuff because that is for people who cogitate, and I wasn't up for that. But it does make me want to get botox now. Maybe. Probably not. But still.

And then, wouldn't you know it, something clicked. Now, I wouldn't know it, because I wasn't thinking about it and was just gliding along, like a happy little water strider that got straight C's in school and can't keep a relationship. Water strider doesn't care. Things were slowly changing in its tiny bug brain, but it's not paying attention.[3]

Level Three forgiveness happened one day when I decided to square up with salads.

Every spring, my mom and I talk about her vegetable patch. My parents planted a gigantic garden because they actually like vegetables. Mom has a big thing for radishes, which are, in my opinion, the sullen teenager of produce. Each phone conversation would be about the influx of tomatoes, green beans, zucchini, and so many radishes. Like, what is it with the radishes, Mom? You are giving that vegetable way too much credit. But as we talk about cucumbers and making pickles and meals that sound like they are composed only of squash, I envy it. She loves vegetables. And I don't.

I like mashed potatoes with butter, ok? I like abundance, remember? And vegetables don't have "when you're done eating this you're gonna push yourself away from the table with a deep contented sigh and say 'that was the best radish of my LIFE'" as part of their marketing plan. They're not gooey and cheesy unless it's broccoli cheese casserole, which I cannot eat because school lunches ruined that for me.

Vegetables always seem like the "we have to" addition to dinner. They're like flood insurance. Nobody wants to get them, and they cause a little resentment.

I realize, too, that there might be some of you reading this who are vegetable lovers, who actually say things like, "Oh! Zucchini!" when dinner starts, but I have never ever said that. Not once. Not in my entire life.

But, one day, I wanted a salad. So, I put some spinach and feta, and a bit of sliced apple in a bowl. I added walnuts. I made a dressing. And I ate it. And it was pretty good.

I ate that salad every day for about two weeks because my brain said it wanted it. I did what my brain asked. And then I noticed that I was feeling a little better and started running again too, all around the same time, and one night I made a squash soufflé thing that was pretty decent.

Oh, and crispy Brussels sprouts with bacon? Those are super good. That one is kind of obvious because it's bacon. I was now following a lot of salad people on Instagram because when you look up one video about salad dressing, then it's a salad onslaught. One guy was making roasted chickpeas, and I tried that, and I liked them too. There was that one time Brian and I had pickled beets at some restaurant and spent about ten minutes talking about how much we loved pickled beets because we are married, and this is the kind of stuff we talk about now.

And then I went and *made* some. I actually planted beets in my backyard and then made my own pickled beets, and I was now Laura Freaking Wilder.

If I'm honest, and this would be the place for it, the beets were a ton of work. They dyed the kitchen red, which was kind of gross, and they produced two jars. I just started buying them after that.

So, Level Three forgiveness was tied to action. Tiny action. *Teeny* tiny action. I decided to have a salad a day. But if I didn't, that's ok. But I would try.

And I did. And I do. I try to eat a salad a day. I also eat radishes, sliced very thinly, on buttered rye bread with a pinch of sea salt. I use really good butter, and I eat it on my pretty plate with the Swedish people on it. It's so good[4] that it made me wonder, what other vegetable is out there, hiding from me? I'm coming for you.

This whole forgiveness thing didn't really change anything. And, also? It changed everything. I still ate in excess sometimes. I still ate so many Blow Pops that I would wake up with a sugary wrapper stuck to me because a good book and way too many Blow Pops were my happy place. I would still find myself digging around late at night for something sweet and resorting to chocolate chips straight from the bag, which didn't really satisfy, and I would shrug and think, "Well, this is stupid but ok." And I skated along, still messing up, and not caring, and making that salad, and wouldn't you know it. I started to feel better about food. Finally. I messed up, and I got better. *At the same time.*

And once in a while, my brain would say, "Hey. I'm bored! Let's have some frozen chimichangas we don't really want," and I would keep reading my book or watching *The Crown* or whatever, and I would say, "No. I think I'll just sit with this for a minute instead." The discomfort would huff, "Hello? C'mon! Let's go!" And I would turn a page and just let the discomfort sit on its haunches until it shifted and scratched itself and got bored too, and then it would lumber off. This is a miracle. It's also recovery. It's progress, not perfection.

It was a tiny, peaceful start.

Notes

1 Mom and Dad, I can hear you. You're saying: But there were egg rolls! Bo Lings' egg rolls! And crab rangoon! We FED you, Dana. This doesn't look good for us. You are not traumatized by appetizers! Get it together! This is what happens when your daughter writes about her past and she gets to consistently throw you under the bus that doesn't have any appetizers in it.

2 #blessed

3 Later in this book, I will talk a whole lot about paying attention to certain things in life, but don't despair readers. Inconsistencies in the book only mean I am complex and nuanced, like an art house film with a drinking problem. All of us humans are complex and nuanced, and as I learn to ignore some things and pay a crap-ton of attention to other things, I beg of you. Just stay with me.

4 You were right, Mom.

Bibliography

1 **Over half of Americans report that they are stressed out:**
Zauderer, Steven (2023, March 9). 67 Workplace Stress Statistics in 2023. https://tinyurl.com/35tkrwxt.

2 **Women do tend to be more aware of the strain in our lives:**
Apa.org. (2023). Stress by Gender. https://www.apa.org/news/press/releases/stress/2012/gender-report.pdf.

3 **Research indicates that women respond to stress more emotionally than men:**
Maisey, Sarah (2023, April 9). Women May Be More Vulnerable to Emotional Overeating, Study Shows. *The National*. https://tinyurl.com/35sr4pez.

4 **And stress is linked to addiction:**
Sinha, Rajita (2008). Chronic Stress, Drug Use, and Vulnerability to Addiction. *Annals of the New York Academy of Sciences* 1141 (1): 105–30. https://doi.org/10.1196/annals.1441.030.

5 **Incidentally, "fake it till you make it" has been scientifically proven to work:**
Robinson, Bryan (2020, August 13). New Study Shows Forming a Simple Smile Tricks Your Mind into a Positive Workday Mood. *Forbes*. https://tinyurl.com/3wd58ner.

10

I Don't Want to Talk About It

Until it's not peaceful. Until I mess it up. Like, I start thinking it's a diet. I start letting the word "thin" float on by. That'll submerge the whole thing.

Some days I go for a run, and I practice good posture, and I smile a lot, and I remember to pray. I remember acceptance and surrender.

Some days I sink. My feelings sit in my chest with a weight. I'm so sad. I try to control things outside of my reach. I forget I'm an addict. My brain buzzes behind my eyes and tells me I am ugly and fat and awful.

I don't write anything. I find myself sitting down a lot. And then, I lie down and start scrolling, and my brain locks me out. I eat all the food. I finish it and then eat some more. I give up on myself by 9 a.m.

Some days I fail. Or, maybe, the day fails me. I can't think about it a lot because if I do, I sink even deeper. I watch a movie at 11 a.m. I sleep. I consider taking a shower, but I am too angry about it—that taking a shower seems like such a hard decision. I yell at the dog. It's a rotten day and I am a rotten person, and that's the day. That's the whole day. Just me and my angry brain.

Some days I just can't seem to remember anything good.

Maybe my meds are off. Or my hormones. Or maybe I did something horrible, and I should be punished. I don't know. I eat more. All the sugar just makes me shaky, and I think, "I'll have to run double miles tomorrow. And I'll do nothing but salads tomorrow. And I'll be nothing but good tomorrow," and I consider these blanket statements as if they are true. I wrap myself up in those blankets and hide.

I just sink.

We all sink some days. It's awful. It's such a mess. Anything good stops making sense, like a clock on the wall that stops ticking.

Nothing is right, and I can't find a center. I can't recalibrate. I consider making a salad now, but that just makes me laugh, but in an awful way, the way bullies laugh at recess.

It's meanness. Some days, I am just so very mean to myself.

And even the next day, I don't wake up knowing the gloom has passed. And I get angrier. And I mess up some more.

But I don't drink. It's a victory that I recognize with a tired "Well. Ok," at the end of the night. I mutter "This too shall pass," and because I like structure, I have a rule. I made the rule long ago; otherwise, I wouldn't remember it in the thick of this.

The rule is: Three days. There are the three wise men, the Three Stooges, and three blind mice, so I can give whatever this is three days. I'll give it three days of hell, and then I'll make a call to Andrea. I promise myself.

So far, it has always lifted by day three. I make a salad. It's one of my favorites, with avocado, red onion, and tomatoes. It's still a Sad Salad, but it has croutons. I feel bruised. I go on a short walk. I feel the sun on my shoulders. My legs feel weak, but I do it anyway. I play fetch with the dog. I remember who I am. I don't eat to the point of feeling ill. I don't hate myself anymore. I remember, finally, and thank you, God, I remember that these awful days are farther apart.

I breathe. I go back to forgiveness. Life is a trip.

11

Parenting Is Impossible

I wrote an entire book about control and perfectionism, and then my children became teenagers.[1] I have been doing my best to help my sons understand addiction, but all those scenarios, the ones I would lecture them about, where they would nod along with their big brown eyes, those scenarios are now here. I want to grab both of my boys, hustle them upstairs to their rooms, and never allow them to leave, but I can't do it. They are taller than I am now. There are logistics.

At times, my anxiety mutters, "You must protect them at all costs! They are doooooomed!" But simultaneously, both boys vex me so much that I long for the 1980s when I could get away with barely parenting them. "Go ride your BMX to the 7–11," I could tell them. "Meet up with sketchy friends and be gone until dinner."

Parenting does not work well in such extremes. Acceptance is key.

When *Bottled* came out, Henry proudly announced to his second-grade class, "My mom is a HUGE alcoholic and she's gonna be on the TODAY show about that!" The second graders all nodded at this, I imagine. Julie, his teacher, probably nodded too, and then made at least four mental notes, as teachers do.

It's true. I am a huge alcoholic and therefore, famous.[2] At least, I was to Henry. At least once. Not so much anymore, because Henry is now fifteen and I'm not even famous-adjacent. This is fine. It's fine. I'm fine.

It's all changing now. Everything. Their voices are different, and they refer to me as "My guy." In sixth grade, one of them handed me this question: "Mom, what does Scotch taste like? Is it like butterbeer?" and I remember thinking,

This is all going to catch up with me at some point. And it has. It's here. Scotch is here. Well, maybe Twisted Tea is here, but it's here.

They no longer ask any questions about addiction. When we watch a movie and someone is drinking and I start in on lecture #437 Why You Shouldn't Do That, they roll their eyes and cut me off with a mutter, "We KNOW. Mom. Stahhhhp." But I forge ahead with the Cliffs Notes, talking fast, and I end up saying "fiftypercentofalcoholicskidsbecomealcoholicstoo" in one breath with an implication of "YOU'RE DOOMED if you touch the stuff" on the side. I'm met with silence. I overshot. One kid looks at the movie screen, ignoring me. The other reaches for his phone, ignoring me. The husband says very little because I'm getting dangerously close to The One Argument We Have Over and Over, and now everyone is irritated. Then, Arnold Schwarzenegger blows somebody up in the movie, and I'm grateful for it.

Brian and Dana's One Argument They Have Over and Over:

Brian: So, then we went to Old Chicago and ate that pizza that isn't really a pizza but is just a drawer of cheese—

Me: But also, you had beer, didn't you?

Brian: Yes. I had a beer.

Me: I knew it. I could smell it. You drank in front of them.

Brian: Yes. I did, and I know we've had this argument about fifty times in our marriage, but here is the part where I act like I've never heard this before.

Me: THIS IS THE PART WHERE WE HAVE THIS ARGUMENT AGAIN, SO YOU CAN ACT LIKE YOU'VE NEVER HEARD THIS BEFORE.

Brian: Stop with the capital letters. I am not a total asshole like you are trying to write me. Hold up.

Me: Too late.

Brian: Ok, I do remember this conversation, but as YOU don't seem to remember, we come to an impasse. This means I still think it's ok to drink occasionally around the boys, and at no point do you say you forbid it because that would be writing you as sort of the asshole, right?

Me:

Brian: So, that's how we left it the LAST time we had this argument, and yet you seem to forget that, and you go full ham every time this comes up. YOU bring it up. And then you pick the fight. I'm totally ok with sitting over here and having a beer that doesn't have all this stuff attached to it.

Me: There is so much attached to that beer. You know that.

Brian: Ok. True. But also, no. If we make a huge deal about drinking with them, then we're going to mess 'em up. Right? I don't attach anything to the beer. It's just beer.

Me: Beer is never just beer! And I don't know. No? Maybe? Uncertainty makes me mad!

Brian: You do remember I grew up—

Me: YES I KNOW. It wasn't a thing. There was no addiction. Your beers were unattached, and your family is normal. Fine! You weirdos.

Brian:

Me: So, if I harp on it, then they might listen and remember and be safe. But you say, don't harp on it, and they might relax and be well-adjusted and safe. So which is it?

Brian: Sort of both? But could we . . . maybe without the fighting?

Me: I don't do *both*. *Gestures at self* I am a one-or-the-other kind of girl. Have you not been married to ME for nearly twenty years?

Brian: Yes. Yes, I really have.

Me: *Slaps hands together* All right. This concludes session #51 of That One Argument We Have Over and Over. Just to wrap up: We've come to a final decision. No drinking ever around them, never ever, or until the next time you have a beer with your pizza, and I freak out about it.

Brian: *Checks calendar* So, in about four or five months or so. Let's get it on the calendar now.

Here's some information that likes to camp out in my brain: children of alcoholics have an increased risk for depression. They can have more challenges with relationships, dealing with their emotions, or needing a sense of control over their world. I see this already in both of my boys, but when I point it out to Brian, he adds helpfully, "Isn't that kind of thing for all teenagers, in general?" This makes my head hurt. I become hyper-vigilant in spurts of energy, but then I just want to go to bed at 8 p.m. and not worry so much. I'm pretty sure menopausal fatigue and hormonal anxiety are contributing to this, but when I point this out to Brian he adds, helpfully, "Isn't that kind of what parenting is like, in general?" and I wander off to find a place to lie down and mutter at him while prone.

And there's my dad telling me, long ago: "Dana. Fifty percent. Fifty percent of children of alcoholics become alcoholics themselves." Math is not uncertain. It's clear-cut. This is an equation, and our family had the right answer, if you can call one dead son and a daughter in recovery out of the four of us, something "right." It was all kinds of wrong, but it sure didn't leave any questions. Children of alcoholics have four times more of a chance of struggling with addiction. It's my father's voice again, telling me I'm already locked in, and my two boys, young and strong and so very loved, are doomed.

I didn't allow myself to think about this much when they were little. I was just trying to stay sober, taking the days in increments, figuring out a wholly new reality that seemed very intent on shifting all the spaces inside me. First, I was emptied out. Then I was filled with a new type of living. It's lovely, all these clean new rooms, but it takes a whole lot of work and sweat and shoving and lifting and moving around. The first year, I scrambled around for new habits. It started with knitting because I desperately needed my hands to have something to hold onto instead of a wine glass. All those wine glasses didn't make room for hobbies, so the clicking of the knitting needles was a new melody—not just a replacement for the wine glass, but a whole new action. A movement. I was a terrible knitter. I made contorted scarves with increasingly tight stitches, so the scarves looked like they were trying to strangle themselves. Eventually, I set the knitting down, storing it in my new empty rooms of sobriety, and found some more space for something like yoga, or making bread. All of this took time, and there were days when my bread turned out like a yeast brick, and I hated it all, hated trying, hated that I couldn't drink wine along with my bread (while knowing that the bread thing would not have a chance after a glass or six), and that's pretty much early sobriety for you.

The boys were little, and I moved through this with them, explaining my absences for meetings and just holing up in my room as "mom's time to get better," and it worked. The boys didn't ask questions. They cuddled anyhow. They watched *Little Einsteins* with me in bed, curled up and happy to have a mom who was not always around, but when she was? She *was*.

There were no questions from them. Mom leaves on Wednesday nights to go to a meeting. What meeting? No clue. No worries. Does it matter? Nope—she'll be there later for cuddles and some *Wild Kratts*, and that's ok. She also makes a lot of cookies because she's baking her way through a lot of mom guilt, and that's awesome.

I mean, probably this is the case. I'm not sure about any of this. I fiddle around with uncertainty. Perhaps my boys will need therapy. Maybe I royally screwed them up. Maybe they have deep fears about abandonment or lack of control, or they feel like they've got to fix it when people get upset. Perhaps my boys are messed up because I was the original messer-upper. I don't know how to put all this into words for them and ask. Should I just say it? "Hey? Are you going to crash and burn someday because your mom did it first? Are you going to fall apart too? Did I do that to you?"

And, what if you die? What if you die at fifty-seven, like my brother did?

These are the thoughts that sometimes drip through and stain the floors in my pretty new rooms. They come at night, usually. They slam into me with assurance and dread, and I think, "Well, Dana, that would be consequences for your actions, wouldn't it?" And I am so grim about it at 3 a.m., hating myself and hating what I did. Grim is so easy in the middle of the night.

Two teenage boys don't ask questions, but they certainly do make me want some solid answers. When you find out your fifteen-year-old was driving around with his buddies at ten at night, and you didn't know, you didn't even know who he was with or when he would be home, because everyone in our house is on a different schedule, it hits differently. You messed up and miscommunicated, and he disappeared for a while, and swirling around in the back of your mind is this soft little sneer, "Anything can happen. Anything. And the odds are stacked against him, so that 'anything' could be really, really bad. And it's *your fault*."

So when the kid gets home at 11 p.m., you yell at him and he yells back, and it's a misery called Parenting: What Not to Do.

But you can't help it.

Here's the hardest thing to admit. It's just the craziest thing. My children are triggers.

There, I said it.

When they were little, I got sober and wrote a book about it, telling moms with little kids that they could do it; that the hectic chaos of having babies while not slipping into a vat of wine each night was possible. It was glorious, the freedom and strength from realizing I could climb what looked like an impossible mountain and live to write about it.

But here's the thing: a recovery mountain doesn't have an official summit. There's no flag at the top with a "You made it!" photo op, and now, I have two sons who might sidle right up next to me on the climb, holding a beer, and say, "Here I am with an explosive device in my hand, and you can't do much about it." When they were little, when the worries would surface as I watched them sleeping, so little with their soft breaths and pudgy feet and impossible eyelashes, I could pray over them and surrender them, but also I could relax a little. No toddler was going to wake up the next morning and say, "The details are sketchy, but my friends want to go stand around in a field and drink warm beer[3] and I'm going to go, even though I told you I was just hanging out playing Fortnite." The toddler is still cute. He likes to sit in puddles and pull off his shoes, and play with worms. You can sit with him, and it's all pretty contained.

Now, the teenager is always moving, and often that movement is on the brink of something, a balance beam between right and wrong, a narrow road, the edge of a glass.

Shame and addiction are highly linked. Any mother reading this right now who suffers from a substance use disorder is rolling her eyes. Of *course* it is. Shame is sticky, like hot tar stuck to the sidewalls of a car. Scrubbing doesn't work. You will deface your nice car. Prying it off is doable, but scratches can happen. Damage piles on damage.

Here are some other descriptors of shame:

It's very detail-oriented.

It's persistent; it likes to hang around.

It's attentive, always watching.

Shame is powerful, strong, and very dependable.

Shame is acutely self-aware.

Ok, now do a little experiment with me. Reread the list above, but substitute the words "Awesome Partner" for the word "Shame," and wow, would you look at that? The most confusing thing about shame is that it's deeply rooted in love.

Breaking up with shame is super hard because you'll second-guess yourself the moment after you yell at it to leave. "Maybe I shouldn't have been so harsh," you think. "Maybe it's not so bad . . . " and shame reliably comes right back, holding a big bouquet of substance, any substance, to numb.

Shame's cyclical tendencies become almost soothing because they're so predictable. Anything predictable, even negatively, scratches some sort of itch in my brain. And, shame's grip keeps women silent. We are the mothers, the nurturers. How could I abandon my child like this? So, we suffer in silence, literally, not self-reporting, not asking for help, not reaching out. The shame of it all keeps us stuck and still.

And here's the absolute crappiest thing about shame: trying to pin it down is so internal and intense that it coaxes me to look outward, to focus on my sons as the antidote for pain. If I can fix *them*, work on *them*, and keep *them* safe, the problem will be solved. Shame gives me something else to look at instead of my sadness. This is shame's ultimate sleight of hand, controlling the room and keeping me in my seat. It's quite a show.

My kids are a show. They are funny and loud, and often there's a fight scene[4] or at least some sort of physical humor on stage. I have applauded them and laughed with them, and cried with them. They are a hit. A spectacle. They're here every night. It's a five-star feature; every day we are together. But shame messes with this and says things like, "They are too good for you. You don't deserve it."

Shame is horrible.

So, enough about that. Because as much as shame likes to catch me up with all my feelings, I am going to admit another triggery truth that's happening right at the same time: My children are also, like, *so annoying.*

This is where guilt sidles in. My sons do things like leave styrofoam cups of congealed Oreo shakes under their beds until they're stuck to the floor. They walk into rooms and scatter a wake of clothes and chip bags, and then leave those rooms completely blind to the floor. The floor does not exist to them even though they walk on it.

They mutter, "Yes, I'm doing it right now" when I ask them to take out the recycling, but they are saying this in a strange monotone tone while completely prone on the couch watching a YouTube video about a guy who yells about Fortnite a lot. I have observed this, for real. A son, sitting on a couch, telling me that he is taking out the recycling *right now*. Has he broken the space/time continuum? Is this *Interstellar*? When prompted about this, he acts incredulous and says things like "Dude I'm GETTING to it," to which part of my brain starts smoking.

They don't get to it.

They are asked to clean the bathroom but completely ignore wiping down the shower, which, in all honesty, is not as gross as the other parts of the bathroom, but still. And when questioned about it, they say, "What? That's the SHOWER. I didn't know you wanted me to clean that. You just said the bathroom," and I want to scream. How do you lecture someone about parts of a house? Do you draw pictures? A PowerPoint?

You make homemade chocolate banana muffins that they loved last week, and one of them says, "Yeah, don't put that in my lunches. They taste like bananas," and you stare down at the muffins and wonder if you can trade your kid for someone who likes bananas.

They shout downstairs at 7:01 a.m. as you are just starting to pour a cup of coffee, "MOM YOU MOVED MY BLACK BASEBALL T-SHIRT THAT LOOKS LIKE EVERY OTHER BLACK T-SHIRT IN THIS HOUSE WHERE IS IT." You might have moved it. You don't know. It's seven in the morning. But you must find it because the baseball team will trade the kid, and the school will fire him if it's not located. Also, all three of you are now late, so the added stress of getting to school on time makes your tired brain kind of seize up into a glommy wad. When the t-shirt is finally located and then both kids are dropped off with a mutter and a door slam, you come home and look down at the cold cup of coffee.

By the way, what is the deal with all the black t-shirts, sports teams? Branch out.

They ask for money and then lose it. They need permission slips to be signed and lose them. They lose sweatshirts, baseball gloves, homework, water bottles,[5] charging cords, and the ability to look at the floor. They constantly work away at the screws that you have tightened that keep the house and life in running order and then shout a lot when things go tilty.

They call you "bruh."

You respond with infinite grace and patience, the mother of all mothers, smiling beatifically and keeping it all together even when they wake you up asking where their underwear is because they have also lost the ability to push buttons on that big white thing in the laundry room. You gently instruct and, most importantly, allow for learning opportunities to keep them responsible for their actions, so they grow up to be mature and fully realized young men of the world.

No, that's total bullshit. You yell at them at 7:02 a.m.

Not all the time. I am the adult after all. But there is a certain voice, a certain whining "MOM" that they utilize that makes my shoulders jump up to my ears, and I hear myself answer it back with a "*WHAT*" that calls their "MOM" and raises it twenty.

Sometimes I remember to pray. I say, "God, help me to be a good mom today. Just give me patience," and then I find myself slamming kitchen drawers, which is anticlimactic because we have those fancy ones that silently slide shut.

About an hour later, these moments turn into congealed cups of guilt. Guilt says, "You did this horrible thing. You should have calmed down. They are never going to realize there is a floor there with all this yelling."

Guilt says, "You did bad."

Shame then comes and sits down, hands you a pillow, and adds, "You **are** bad."

All of this happens before eight in the morning.

I deeply love my children, and sometimes I want to leave them somewhere else. This type of pendulum behavior is a common trope among parents, but it can work differently when addiction is part of one of the parents. Ok, it's me. I'm the problem; it's me.

I have an addictive personality, so guilt and shame crouch in my head and fester, and then transform into something else: triggers.

The term "trigger" is thrown around a lot these days, sometimes legitimately, or sometimes not. I once had a student in my college class write me a five-paragraph email about how my essay's due date was triggering her, and I wanted to respond with a meme of Inigo Montoya saying, "You keep using that word. I do not think it means what you think it means."

When I first got sober, I figured triggers would happen. I was ready. Triggers take you back to drinking, so for me, that was any person, place, or thing that reminded me of white wine. Dinnertime preparation? Six p.m. trigger. People laughing and drinking outside a local bar, the condensation misting their pretty glasses (and yes, I could spy that just walking by. I was hyper-aware): communal trigger.

Sometimes a song that leaned heavily into a time I was drinking—for me, it was Nat King Cole's *The Christmas Song*—took me right back to cozy mulled wine or Irish cream. Nat King Cole became a festive trigger, which is also a really good way to ruin a lovely song. Thanks, alcoholism.

Triggers are just stimuli, and the brain's limbic system responds. It's completely normal;

If someone pokes you, you flinch. Triggers poke, and the brain flinch-remembers, and all of a sudden, Nat King Cole has all this stuff attached to him. I worked on it. I avoided people, places, and things that sounded alarms. I became weird and avoided happy Christmas music. I didn't drive by my favorite haunt, a liquor store, for months in early sobriety. I didn't attend a wedding for a full year.

And then I enrolled in an intense sort of exposure therapy: I had children.

Children are triggers. They stupefy and nullify things that you thought were important. They come with their own exhaustion starter packs, and they upgrade on this constantly. But dang if I didn't think that as I increased my years of sobriety, perhaps their ability to make me lean back into addictive behavior would dissipate. More sobriety, more strength. That sort of thing. And yes, I didn't drink today, even though the same pair of dirty underwear still remains on the bathroom floor and has been so for at least three days, because I refuse to pick it up. It's become a thing now. A social experiment.

They trigger me. I don't drink anymore. But I eat. Or scroll. Or falter in a whole lot of process-addiction ways, but honestly? The hardest part about all of this is just admitting it. The fact that they trigger me *triggers me*. They poke at my feelings and remind me how nice it would be to numb out.

It's shameful. I love them both so much. How can I admit to such a thing?

And here we go on the whole shame-cycle ride, once again. Until my husband walks up, picks up a dirty utensil on the counter, and asks me this: "Why is this spoon here?" and oh! THEN I remember:

People we love the most also annoy the crap out of us. Stitch that on a pillow. And annoyance, when sculpted by the alcoholic brain that is mine, often leans back into how I used to soothe myself. Being triggered by someone I love is ok. It's just not ok to *act* on it. So, as the parenting life continues for me, I learn to pay attention. I say the serenity prayer a lot. I breathe. I practice acceptance. I ask for forgiveness.

I text my older son:

Me: I'm sorry I was cross.

My son: u ight.

I think that means I'm all right. Let me look it up on Urban Dictionary. I pay attention to these new things, all the newness of teenagers. We embark into the "judgmental NOW" of teenage boy brains, meaning they make snap judgments on everything, like they're constantly flinging little judgmental ninja stars at anything moving. Charlie judges our cat Lucy. Lucy is small and soft and gray and just about the most adorable thing moving around in our house, but he judges her. "She's *loud*," he says witheringly, as she sits like a perfect little cat potato on his bed. How can he say this? Lucy is a gray fluff of near perfection. And I've never even heard her meow. Not once. Does he not understand volume levels? If that level of bias is already occurring with her, what does he think about me, the alcoholic mom who isn't cute at all? I can't curl up like a small loaf and blink slowly at them. I don't have a chance.

This is normal. This is all part of the process. My teenage sons' brains are set on a circling wheel when it comes to empathy or feelings. They process a lot with their amygdala, the emotions' call-center of the brain. Their prefrontal cortex is still basically offline; it's last in line to fully develop, to fully sync up with all the other parts of the brain. I should remember this in the heat of the moment, but when it's the heat of the moment, my amygdala is on full steam too, so it's an amygdala smackdown.

The boys have judged me for standing too close, for breathing, for asking what "rizz" means. I still don't know what it means, but I dropped it because I couldn't take the withering looks. At home, my sons are The Plastics. I have asked, and their teachers report they are not like this at school. They have friends; their teachers say they are nice, and they don't wear pink on Wednesdays. But I'm the mom, and this morning when I asked one of them what time he had to leave, he said "I TOLD you" with such languid pain that I felt bad he had such an addled mother.

Ok. Granted, this is normal. All parents feel this unless their children are nice. But ultimately, I fear their scary judgey powers might land on my recovery. Do they know more than alcoholism? Will they file addiction away as just a weakness? The addled mother. The silly addict. They'll be smarter than that, surely, because they already know ALL the things. Once, when I was telling them about their birth story, Charlie interrupted me to correct me on my C-section, so he does, in fact, know all there is.

And damn, if that wasn't me. When I knew my dad went to Wednesday night meetings, and I knew that my brother also struggled, I filed it under "Well, I know better than that," and we saw how that worked out. I try to tell them this. I try to come up with a logical and compelling argument, and I try and try, and I don't know . . . I don't KNOW if it's getting through. I just don't KNOW for sure.

Being triggered by Dotties Liquor store that I pass every time I pull into the grocery parking lot is one thing. Being triggered by someone I love and am actively caring for is another.

"New territory. New territory," I mutter, as I help one kid learn to parallel park and another to traverse a first date. One of my triggers just started shaving. What is happening? College names are being thrown around in casual conversation. Flashes of anger, sadness, and glee swirl around us like dramatic dust motes, and I want to grab hold of both sons and discuss all these new feelings like a useless mom-therapist, but the dust motes just float through my fingers, up to their rooms to FaceTime their friends.

Sometimes my boys get quiet, and I ask myself: Is it dangerous? Or is it just a teenager? I go up and sit on the beds and we talk a little. Or, I force myself to wait. It's all so delicate, which is saying a lot for two humans who regularly strew underwear and belch a lot.[6]

I get still. I get afraid. I think, "The main reason you drank was because of depression." I go to the bottom of the stairs and look up, wondering what to ask that will unlock it all and give me the answers I long for. The kid is upstairs looking at a screen. I can hear him talking to Henry. He could be enjoying *The Mandalorian*.[7] (Hey! I'll watch it with you! I had asked, trying to be enthused about another Star Wars spinoff with a lot of backstory and beige clothing. He responded, "Nah. Ima do my own thing.") Or, he could be depressed. Or both?

I read articles about teenage depression. I talk to friends. I dive into videos about reactive parenting and how it lowers cognitive abilities in children. I try to calm down. I also make plans. I pray. I say: I will not react; I will gather information. This makes me feel like I'm trying to be Brian. He is a gatherer of information. He doesn't overreact. He asks a lot of questions, but then I remember him asking me about the spoon on the counter and think his methods might be a bit too specific and too annoying.

I breathe. I say, "It's grace and nothing more." I still pray over them in the night while they're sleeping. Boys, when you read later, yes, it's me. I'm the mother, it's me. I come in and watch you sleep, and you will need to let me do it, or we'll be back at yelling. I yell anyway. It's impossible.

Here are some other impossible things: Covid made me crazy with worry. Our country's political situation makes me want to cry, especially in the car, for some reason. Why does driving always make me think of politics?

My parents are getting older. Our taxes are due. Brian and I got married in our late thirties, so if my children ever get married and have kids, I'll be too old to know it. Blueberries cost so much now that I have started saying things like "Don't eat all the fruit!" to my younger son, who loves fresh fruit and would probably choose it over packaged cookies, and here I am fruit-shaming him. I hide blueberries in the vegetable drawer. Social media keeps sending me videos of neighbors being mean to each other for some reason, and I stare, transfixed by the awfulness of humans.

Six months ago, I had a cancer scare, and it was also impossible. I had no control. There was so much waiting. And when it was finally decreed that I was in the clear, I didn't exactly feel happy, just shell-shocked.

My cat Bob and my dog Hosmer both died within a few months of each other, and I think I can't take anymore leaving pets. We got another dog, a

German Shepherd, who eats the house, but in a cute way. And then, I watched a documentary about an octopus.

The octopus is a mom (a momoctopus?) and spends months caring for her tiny eggs. She never leaves them, not even to eat. Then, they are born, and she dies. We see her carried away in the jaws of a shark.[8] It's so awful. There's no warning. She was the best mom ever, and look. Look what happened.

Everything is impossible. We love things, and we fear how much we love. The documentary is called *My Octopus Teacher,* and I watched the ending with tears streaming down my face. I'm not sure I want to learn what that octopus can teach me. It's all so hard.

Fear and learning don't mix. It puts both the teachers and the students into a state of fight or flight, and that keeps us in amygdala territory—frozen in our feelings and poised for conflict. We don't process. We don't think. I remember my fourth-grade teacher insisting that I grasp a long-division problem long before I was emotionally prepared. At the start of our relationship, long division was just terrible to me. And the teacher, whose name I will never forget, but for the sake of her family I will call Mrs. Grim, would lean over me, her halitosis and harshness lingering over my head just in my blind spot, and she would sigh and say, "Just THINK, Dana. Just think HARDER," as if I could squeeze the long division out of me, which is gross.

I learned long division the **next** year from Mr. Amthauer, who played guitar and sang to us, and we could all belt out the chorus to Paul Simon's *50 Ways to Leave Your Lover* even though we didn't understand what was going on in the song.

I'm learning to parent teenagers. They're learning to **be** teenagers. In there, mixed in with deadly and also strengthening properties, is my recovery. It's a whole new world.

And also, it's an old one. Because it simply takes it back to acceptance and surrender, which is a lot after school drop-off at eight in the morning, but here we are (Figure 11.1).

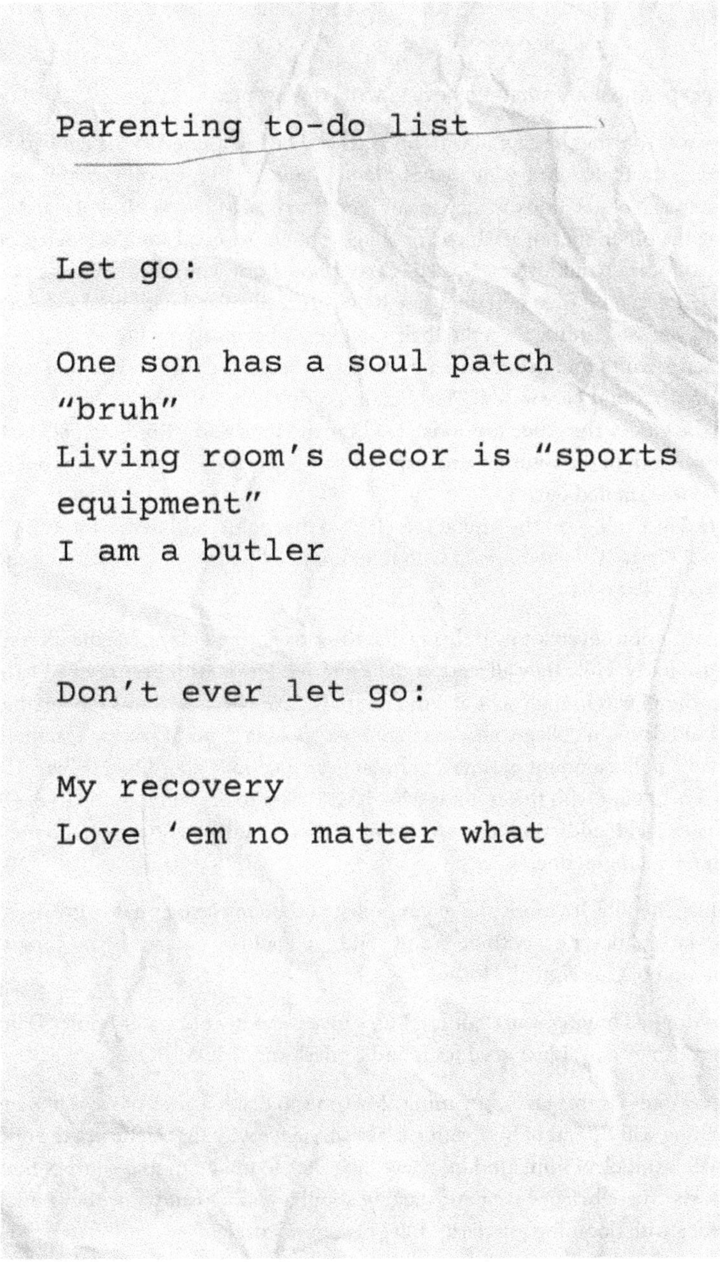

```
Parenting to-do list


Let go:

One son has a soul patch
"bruh"
Living room's decor is "sports
equipment"
I am a butler


Don't ever let go:

My recovery
Love 'em no matter what
```

Figure 11.1 *Do Your Best*

Notes

1 I did get permission from both boys to write this chapter.

2 Henry was touring the capital with his class and he mentioned to the guide that I had a book in the State Library. *Bottled: A Mom's Guide to Early Recovery* was nominated as a Kansas Notable Book, which means I am famous. My book kind of stands out among the other offerings, which are mainly about historical stuff, or poetry, or a guide to Kansas wildflowers. *Bottled* is about how I drank my face off while parenting small children and then quit doing so. It doesn't really blend with books about Dwight Eisenhower. So, finding it on the shelf would have been easy, right?

When Henry's tour group entered the library, he texted me: "hey dont u you have a book in here" and I answered! "Yes! Pix or it didn't happen!" and that's when he spoke up to the guide. The guide just looked at him and then said, "Riiiiight. Let's just go look at the artwork in the rotunda" and my moment to once again prove how cool I am to my son was snuffed out.

One day, I will go to the capital myself, find that guide, and have a total "Big mistake. HUGE." *Pretty Woman* moment with him, but in a literary way and without the wad of hundred dollar bills.

3 Honestly, I don't even know if that's what the kids do these days. Maybe it's some sort of house party while they all stare at their phones. Fields with beer seemed to be the thing when I was in high school. I did not participate because I was too terrified of my dad. I did drink in college but even then I wasn't a big drinking mess. Yea, me! Instead, I waited a polite amount of time and became an alcoholic after I had babies. There are layers of guilt with this but it is what it is. Trying to explain it to folks who don't have issues with addiction feels awful sometimes. Thanks for sticking with me in this chapter. It's a tough one.

4 Not, like, literally. It's more like stage combat and there's usually a dog involved. Whoever said never act with dogs and children would be amazed by the long-running production of Our Nutball House.

5 I have stopped buying water bottles. I now give them my old water bottles from 2015 that say things like "I just need Jesus and Coffee" and "MOM BOSS."

6 I'm sorry but—is this just a boy thing? My son can drink a glass of ice water and then something will rip out of him with such baritone ferocity that it startles the dog. The dog will just look at him, kind of in awe, like she's found a kindred spirit of bodily functions. These belches are new; starting about a year ago and now they punctuate my existence with booming regularity. Oh brave new world.

7 Later I found out that Pablo Pascal was the Mandalorian and so I started watching it with my boys whether they liked it or not, because: Pablo Pascal.

8 Uh, spoiler alert? Sorry. It's still a really good documentary if you're willing to let an octopus mess with your head.

Bibliography

1. **Children of alcoholics have an increased risk for depression:**
Murray, Emily (2021, September 27). How Growing Up with Alcoholic Parents Affects Children. *Addiction Center*. https://www.addictioncenter.com/alcohol/growing-up-alcoholic-parents-affects-children/.

2. **Children of alcoholics have four times more of a chance of struggling with addiction:**
AACP (2019, May). Alcohol Use in Families. https://tinyurl.com/3w9z69kj.

3. **Shame and addiction are highly linked:**
Rahim, Masuma, and Robert Patton (2015). The Association between Shame and Substance Use in Young People: A Systematic Review. *PeerJ* 3: 737. https://doi.org/10.7717/peerj.737.

4. **And, shame's grip keeps women silent:**
Stringer, Kristi L., and Elizabeth H. Baker (2015). Stigma as a Barrier to Substance Abuse Treatment among Those with Unmet Need: An Analysis of Parenthood and Marital Status. *Journal of Family Issues* 39 (1): 3–27. https://doi.org/10.1177/0192513x15581659.

5. **Triggers poke, and the brain flinch-remembers:**
Godreau, Jeanette (2024, February 16). Emotional Triggers: Why They Matter & How to Manage Them Effectively. *Mindful Health Solutions*. https://mindfulhealthsolutions.com/emotional-triggers-why-they-matter-how-to-manage-them-effectively/.

6. **They process a lot with their amygdala, the emotions call center of the brain:**
Monroe, Jamison (2018, October 23). The Facts about Teen Brain Development. *Newport Academy*. https://www.newportacademy.com/resources/mental-health/teen-brain-development/.

7. **... reactive parenting and how it lowers cognitive abilities in children:**
Li, Pamela (2022, February 23). "Reactive Parenting—What It Is & How to Overcome." *Parenting for Brain*. https://www.parentingforbrain.com/reactive-parenting/.

8. **... I watch a documentary about an octopus on Netflix:**
Ehrlich, Pippa, and James Reed (2020, September 7). My Octopus Teacher. *IMDb*. https://www.imdb.com/title/tt12888462/.

Part III

Dessert

12

Stand Up

I have done stand-up comedy twice now. I remained alive after both incidents.

Saying Yes to these gigs was like early sobriety. I was scared. I tried not to overthink it. I ended up talking a lot in front of a group, and I just kept showing up. "Keep coming back, kid," stand-up chortled at me. "It works if you work it!"

In terms of risky behavior, putting yourself behind a microphone that amplifies both your jokes and your breathing while the audience thinks, "Make me laugh or I'll get out my phone" is pretty high-level stuff. I'm willing to suggest that anyone who thinks otherwise go ahead and sign up for the amateur night at any comedy shop around, and then report back to me. I'll wait right here.

The whole thing started with a text from my friend Jeremy:

I'm doing a comedy show in my backyard.

You should do it too.

And I said *Yes.*

That was weird.

The Backyard Comedy Show was created to celebrate Jeremy's birthday, and it also, organically, was a sort of celebration of getting through the pandemic. Jeremy had been doing some amateur comedy gigs for a while, and he invited a friend of his, Jaron Myers, as the headliner.[1] Jeremy and I would be the warm-ups. It was outside. It was no big deal. It was all just a bit of fun. A few years prior, I had briefly contemplated doing stand-up because it might hone my "craft" and because writing funny is hard. There's timing, and there's hyperbole, and sometimes being funny feels like it's going to kill me, which is hyperbole but not all that funny. But then I decided not to get crazy, and that "honing my craft" just sounded snooty, so I let stand-up comedy go. I didn't want to be scared and snooty at the same time.

But this time, I said yes. Again. Very weird.

As is our way with summer, our family likes to take our calendar and stuff it as full as we possibly can. The boys had tennis and baseball camps. Both kids had church camp, and Charlie was going to Denver for a special STEM nerd camp that entailed getting Covid tests and endless paperwork because he's gifted and makes us do annoying things about it. There was our family vacation one week before the show. I had a traveling speaking gig two weeks prior to that. Additionally, I was still in the throes of numerous doctors' visits to help solve the mysteries of Dana.

So, saying Yes to something entirely new and time-consuming shouldn't be a problem, right? Because that's logical.

What I'm trying to say here is that I don't know why I said Yes to Jeremy. Everything in my life at that point was pointing toward a big fat NO. It was terrifying to even think about making people laugh for twenty minutes straight. Who does that?[2] Why would someone try to do that? Also, I wasn't feeling particularly funny. Life was stressful, and I had a lot of weirdness medically going on. I could go up there and overshare about the weirdness, but I would assume there would only be crickets as a response. Like, literal crickets.

But, as I started working on my lines, this weird automatic Yes thing started reminding me of something else. There was that one time that I decided to say Yes to getting sober.

You see, I didn't really *want* to get sober. Not at all. I loved alcohol. The ritual and the feelings, and all the time it consumed, were such a blast for me. (Not really, but I kept trying to remember it that way, and my brain was pretty pickled by that point.) Quitting it also seemed like a big fat no. My calendar was already packed. I had drinking penciled in every day. Plus, it seemed impossible.

But yet, on a summer day in 2011, I weirdly just said Yes. And I stopped.[3] I stopped drinking. That makes it sound simple, and you *know* it wasn't. But I said Yes to it. I was shaky and ill, and I wasn't doing much thinking. My prefrontal pulled down the blinds, and my motor skills maneuvered me around. I slept. I woke. I drank water. I found keys. I drove. I entered a building. I sat down. I cried. I cried some more. I kept crying. I spoke briefly. I let people pat me on the back. I stood in a circle. I held the hands of total strangers. I prayed. I cried more. I found keys. I wobbled out to the car. I drove home. I ate something. I slept.

These types of surprising Yes's in my life—the ones without much thinking, that originated with just putting one foot in front of the other—they amaze me. For the most part, they've been good. They've served me. I never thought about whether I should marry Brian or not. I just knew we were locked in.[4] I didn't think about it much. I mean, it's just a life-changing decision to pair my entire existence with another human being until one of us dies; what's the big deal? I also didn't think about quitting birth control. I just proceeded. Brian and I talked about it briefly, and I got freaked out and changed the topic to sports. But one night, I just took the little plastic container with all those pills and threw them away. I didn't make a list of pros or cons, and wondered if it was time. I think I got pregnant the next week, which was a bit dramatic, uterus. I hadn't even told Brian that I was not taking the pill anymore. So, I sprung it on him. He said, "Awesome!" and we bought a car seat, and I had a baby. About eighteen months after Charlie, I did the same thing again. I had suffered for months with postpartum depression. It lifted, and I didn't think about it, and we got pregnant and whammo, there was Henry. I kept moving forward. It's kind of dumb, really. It's kind of risky, all this non-thinking about things. Thank goodness I don't much care about thrill rides or I'd probably attempt some sort of extreme sport in there, but my kind of not-thinking never involved heights.

Ok, I know. I know this makes me sound pretty loosey-goosey or willy-nilly, and that doesn't match up with my perfectionistic, List Czar qualities. But in these cases? I knew that if I DID think about it too much, none of the good things would have happened.

It was like my brain sidled out of the way, so my soul could stand up for me. My soul has my back. Always. It's a good soul.

Of course, this weird yes thing has also worked against me. I didn't think much about my relapse either. But really? My relapse wasn't saying yes to anything. It was only saying no to my own life.

Daily, humans say yes to others six times more than they say no. But I'm wondering, how often do we say yes to *ourselves*? It's easy to help someone in a "Hey, can you come over and help me move my sofa" kind of way. But how often do we automatically affirm those needs in our lives that are scary and hard, but will make our souls deeply happy?

I'm fairly good at moving sofas. But for a while, after *How to Be Perfect Like Me* was published, I succumbed to sadness, and I became very good at nixing my soul. I'd lost my way. And, honestly? I'm not sure doing stand-up comedy was going to make me happy. It was kind of terrifying. But I think it was a *gate* to happy.

When the boys were younger, Brian and I attempted a Yes Day exactly twice. We did this because Jennifer Garner[5] told us to, and I do what Jennifer Garner says, ok? At the beginning of the fateful day, we gave both boys a few rules (no trips to Vegas, no ponies[6]) and then said, "To everything else, we will say 'Yes.'" We did this because I wanted to prove, once and for all, that I was a keeper. Besides, they had lived a hard life of impoverishment and denial,[7] and excess equals happiness, right?

Do you know? Yes Day just ended up being expensive, and we were all kind of tired about halfway through. We have not attempted it since, because Yes Day in this economy would mean choosing between it and health care.

But I have wondered about it. If I gave myself a Yes Day, to just grab big handfuls of all the things and experiences I wanted, would I know? Would I know what I should say Yes to?

I think that's why stand-up was such a gift. It was terrifying and true, and it woke me up.

The night of the performance was extremely sticky because this is Kansas, and that's our thing. It was early August. The air was thick with humidity and mosquitoes. I wore an itchy shirt, and sweat gathered in the folds of my stomach and my armpits and ran down into a soggy reservoir in the back of my underwear. There was no breeze. Jeremy has lots of friends, and I have some, and they all seemed to show up that night, lawn chairs in tow. I've written funny stuff before; I'd even won some awards for it, but people can just read whenever they like. They're not sitting right in front of me, waiting for me to entertain them. I was scared. The sun set, and I considered sneaking out. Instead, Jaime, Jeremy's wife, found me over by the lemonade. Jaime is perky. She's got this brilliant smile and a soft husky voice that tells you "I'm here for it! All of it!" and she grinned big at me. "You ready?"

I shook my head. "Jaime, I am so nervous."

She shook her head right back at me. "Nah. You're gonna rock it." Jaime's smile is the kind that goes right up to her eyes, and her eyes were telling me she believed I could rock it. Jaime is not a delusional person, I don't think. So, it helped.

I am not sure if I rocked it or not. Jaime introduced me, I walked out to applause, and I started.

"But Dana," the judgey one that is reading this says, "It's just your friends. It's just a backyard. *It's not that big of a deal.*"

It's not. I totally understand this comment because my judgey brain was right along with you, thinking that my fear was silly.

It was too hot. My makeup was sliding off. And I stood up, under a couple of lights rigged just for the occasion, and I started with a joke about how every good comedian knows to mess with the mic stand. Once you mess with a mic stand, fuss with its cord, and adjust the height a bit, you have established yourself as the real deal.

People laughed.

At least, that's what Brian told me. I don't know. I tend to block things out. But all in all, the set went well, and I have the video to prove it.

And then I did it again, the very next year, because I wanted to make sure I had heard that right.

But it changed me. I stood up.

Did you know that a straight posture helps us remember good memories more often than bad ones? The study I read used defining terms such as "collapsed" or "slumped," which block out the good stuff. Even the words describing lumpy posture sound sad.

I stood up. I found a way.

I found a way on that hot summer night to a new place. I got brave and walked out there, right up to a mic and some friends and a whole lot of jokes about my husband.

Every day, when my son Henry arrives home from school, we like to have a few minutes together where he tells me about gym class. This has been a repeated point of conversation between us since he was in kindergarten. Gym class specializes in all the sorts of games that would terrify me. I did ask once, "Hey, do they make you climb that huge, horrible rope up to the ceiling?" to which his brows furrowed in confusion.

"No. Like, to escape? What? Wait. Why? Why would anyone do that?" and I felt so seen. Instead, Henry's physical education teacher liked games called scatterball, which Henry referred to as "dodgeball but you know, like scattered," and various contortions of basketball, in which Henry regularly features himself as the Lebron James of the bunch. Henry is four feet tall and a scrawny white kid from Kansas, so the comparison is a stretch. But not in his mind. Home from a long day in the trenches of middle school, he'd walk into the kitchen, drop his backpack, his lunch bag, his cello, and about four other things, and then he would begin the recap. Every day, I heard about the magical swishy things he did with a ball and a hoop.

"Moms, I was a straight-up GOAT. FACTS, yo," he would exclaim as I fed him cinnamon toast and nodded a lot. "'N vem I just SWHOOOSSSSHHH" he garbled with his mouth full "'N it was ALLLL" and he would stand up straight, crumbs scattering, and extend both arms out wide, turning his head to the side in a perfect pose of graceful glory, a la Megan Rapinoe at the World Cup. I would almost applaud. It was a beautiful thing. This little seventh-grade punk and his tilted head, arms flung wide stance: it was greatness at the kitchen island.

Right now, as I'm writing this, I stop and stand up, perfectly still and straight, arms wide, head turned, my eyes turned to the horizon. A smile curves my lips. I take a deep breath.[8] My dog Rey trots over and looks concerned. But I'm kind of sure that stand-up was a start. It was a tiny, sweaty start.

If I feel under scrutiny, like I'm on a stage and my audience is waiting for me to dazzle them, a part of my brain can threaten to shut down. It's called the inferior parietal cortex, which is the most fitting name ever, as inferiority is its vibe. It controls those tiny little movements in our lips, our tongue, even our facial expressions, and when we are performing, for example, as a stand-up comic, it can just . . . stop working. This is where the expression "tongue-tied" comes from. It's why I can't take a decent headshot (I'll wait right here while you go check my headshot at the back of the book). My friend Erica has been taking my headshots since *Bottled* came out, nearly ten years ago. She's been with me through three books, an entirely new hair color, and so many weight fluctuations. But she's never been able to get me to smile without looking like I'm remembering to schedule a colonoscopy. She's very kind about it. She'd shoot about five hundred pictures, peer down at her camera monitor, and her brow would just wrinkle the teensiest bit, and then she'd say, "Yes. Well. Let's just get a few more over here," and then approach, move one small piece of hair, and take more pictures. I'd get a cramp. I'd overthink. My smile would get more and more chipmunky, and that doesn't even include all the chins. Don't even get me started on all the chins that would show up to these photo shoots.

Inevitably, we would find one photograph out of the five hundred that sort of worked. A lot of times it was one of the photos I didn't know she was taking because she learned to be stealthy. If I started to pose, my face would go weird and double-chinned like a chipmunk. Perhaps the headshot for this book will have me standing tall, hands on hips, an imaginary cape fluttering in the background in my own superhero pose. If not, just know that it took about five hundred shots to get you this one, so you're welcome. Writing is pain.

Stand-up comedy led me to fulfill a dream I'd had since *Bottled* came out— being able to say: "And thank you for coming to my TED talk."

When I finally got the official "Congratulations! We think you have an idea worth spreading!" email, I called my mother.

I was proud of this achievement. I'd been applying for over a year for a TEDx opportunity. I made it to the final stages a few times, only to be told, "We really like what you have to say, but we regret to inform you . . ." One of the curators encouraged me this way: "I am sure you will do a TED talk one day. Just not this one." Rejection made me slump, but I kept applying. I kept trying. And, when I got the final YES it was a really big deal.

"So. Who's Ted?" my mom asked.

"It's not a who, it's a thing," I countered. "TED talks are like these . . . talks that people give . . . " This sounded lame. "You know! Brene Brown? Everybody's heard that one . . . "

"Renee Brown? No. I thought you said it was Ted."

The conversation kind of spiraled out from there. I still don't think my parents know what a TED talk is, and that's ok. I didn't even mention the TEDx thing. Not because it was a step down from the illustrious TED stage, but because I'm pretty sure "FedEx" would come up. There will be video footage of my talk at some point, and then they can watch that, see the big red TED letters, and still not know what I was doing.

But, I did it. I did a TEDx talk up there, with those big red letters.

And I spoke about being invisible.

Actually, the topic was about my hair. I had gone gray back in 2018, and I wasn't prepared for how monumental this would be to others around me. I still field questions and compliments about my hair color, mainly from women my age. Due to my dad's genes[9] I've been graying since my twenties. But, for me, a weird side effect during this hair thing was occasionally feeling invisible. This was discombobulating. Gray hair seemed to be an entrance into obscurity. It felt like I was pushing up to the bar of life and being ignored, which doesn't make a whole lot of sense since bars aren't my thing anymore. I didn't want to pound on a bar counter and say, "Hey! I'd like a La Croix! I'm over here!" Sometimes it felt easier to just slink away. I wasn't imagining this. Invisible Women Syndrome is a researched phenomenon, where women report that once they reach the age of fifty, they feel left out or passed over by society. Women "of a certain age"[10] are underrepresented in the media. We're left out of clinical trials and medical research, both for our gender and our age. And, pretty much ALL women will go through the wild experience of menopause, yet the physical and mental ramifications of menopause are **still** under-researched.

There were times when my gray hair and I threatened to give in. I'd wake up and walk into the bathroom at 6 a.m. only to be startled by this white-haired woman in the mirror. She looked a bit wrinkled, and her hair was floating around her face, and oh, wait, that was me. My hair changed texture when I let the gray come in, so now it is thick and wavy, reminiscent of a witch over her cauldron, with long tresses and even longer incantations. Or, perhaps that's just the lighting in the bathroom. For a split second in the morning, Broomhilda in the mirror is a bit of a shocker.

But for a split second, when I had brown hair in the mirror, I would forget I was forty. Or, for a split second, some twelve years ago, I would forget I was a mom. For a split second, I'd still feel eighteen on some mornings, or at least twenty-two.[11] And I'd hear The Talking Heads in my own head, asking "How did I get here?"

But, until now, the weirdness with the mirror had always been a quick short-circuit, and then a realization of blessing. My marriage: a blessing. Two sons: crazy blessings.

But old age? Gray Hair? The wrinkles around my eyes? Blessings? It catches me up, and I stare harder, thinking, "Here it is—the old age you always thought happened to others. It's here now and it's YOU," and I have to admit, I don't feel particularly blessed. We've been told by the beauty industry and their endless "anti-aging" mantras that the woman in the mirror is a problem to be dealt with, with expensive creams or needles or surgery. She must be fought off. And yes, it is still called a "beauty" industry. We must not get old, but if we have to, we must have the good manners to do it pretty.

I want to shrug it off, don the feminist mantle of imperviousness to all of this, but also, I miss the beauty part. I miss seeing her—that younger girl with her long lashes. Where did my eyelashes go? My eyebrows are sparse, and my eyelashes don't droop with doe-eyed splendor anymore with a swipe of mascara. Now, they are a bit stubby, and sometimes I can't see well enough to swipe mascara without hitting my eyelid, and jeez getting old is sometimes such a pain in the ass. This is a lot to process at 6 a.m. in a mirror, and I kind of miss the prettier, younger, easier version of me. Sometimes I miss her a lot.

But then I remember she was kind of a mess, and I settle down.

I was so afraid at twenty. I was afraid of being alone. I didn't know how to do it and thought it was a death sentence. In my thirties, I was afraid I'd never get married. And then, I was afraid of becoming a parent. Fearful living was exhausting. I clattered around in three-inch heels a lot back then, too. Ridiculous. All the plumage that was involved. It was such a lot of work.

People fear public speaking more than death, which seems a bit dramatic. They fear it even more than spiders or heights, which is a tough one for me. I speak regularly about my books, and I have been an English teacher for some twenty years, so public speaking was never really a big deal.

But then I said Yes to a TEDx talk.

When I started to prepare for this, I hadn't considered one basic stipulation: I needed to fully memorize about twenty minutes of material and then be able to relate it to an audience in a captivating way. There was a bit of a snag here: my menopausal brain was steeped in brain fog. Like, all the time. Either that, or I have just become incrementally dumber as I have gotten older, but we're going with menopause. Brain fog was one of my biggest issues with menopause symptoms. I would wake in the morning with a literal heaviness behind my eyes and an inability to focus on tasks or remember obligations. It was daunting, but I've always been a big believer in the power of a top-notch list to tackle the day, so my lists and I made the best of it.

I could not make a list for my TEDx adventure. I could not have a teleprompter or, if we're going old school, a sweaty handful of notecards. I could only have me, my brand new pink suit, and my poor, tired brain. Oh, and also, I have ears that constantly buzz and screech, so that wasn't helping either.

"Aw, poor little TEDx Dana," simpers my inner bitchy Dana. "You asked for this. Now suck it up and memorize like you've never memorized before." And I would try, because bitchy Dana had a point. I wrote and rewrote my speech. I worked on sections. I doused it with so many mnemonic devices that the entire talk was one giant acronym.[12] I gritted my teeth and just tried to memorize HARDER. "Think! Dana! Think HARDER!"

I bet you know where I'm going with this.

Everything was going alright until the day of the talk. This is because I love suspense. That morning, I started to walk through my presentation one more time, just a quick little peek at it, and I couldn't remember my lines. I started with a small bobble in the introduction, then I accidentally switched two dates on some research, and then I started leaving out whole chunks. It's like my speech was slowly falling apart in my lap, like nachos in the car, and all I could do was keep trying to nibble.

Around 1 p.m. I found myself on the bed in my Airbnb, staring up at the ceiling, in a kind of horror. My friends kept texting me things like "We're on our way!" and "So super excited!" I wanted to throw up. This was a big mistake. I had made a horrible mistake. I was trying to give a talk tonight about aging, and my aging had decided to sabotage the whole thing.

That's when Brian showed up. Brian often shows up right at the crux of things, and when he does, he is always massively unaware of creeping dread. It's like he's colorblind to the stuff.

I kind of envy him.

He brought in his five bags of stuff[13] for his one-day stay, and then he started scavenging for snacks. I was on the bed, soft and limp, like I'd had a small stroke. The day before, I had participated in one of my favorite speaking-gig traditions by wandering through a Trader Joe's and buying all of their snacks. Snacking is Brian's love language, and he was pretty excited. He jumped up on the bed, with an armful of peanut butter cups and quinoa cheese crunchies, and asked, "So, how you doin'? You ready?"

And then I did a weird thing. I reached over, grabbed the crunchies, and said, "There are mango mochis in the freezer. Also, I got that buffalo chicken dip you like." I didn't tell him. Maybe I should have told him, but instead, I ate some mochi and said, "I sent you about fourteen TikToks at two a.m. last night. Wanna watch them with me?" Brian never says no to this. He might, inwardly, but he always says yes outwardly, and I scooched over and put my head on his shoulder, and he dialed up the fourteen TikToks. Most of them were about cats. He occasionally chuckled. Then, we took a nap.

At about three o'clock, I got up, took a shower, and started to get ready. I put on my fabulous pink suit coat. I still said nothing about my brain freeze. I was on autopilot. I swiped on mascara without poking my eyes. I uncapped my speaking lipstick, Mac's Ruby Woo, leaned into the mirror, and carefully applied it. Ruby Woo is Wonder Woman lipstick. It's here to save the day.

Brian was puttering about and asked me if he should wear the purple Hawaiian shirt or the red one, and I realized something. Brian kind of makes me feel like Wonder Woman. I was currently standing before him with no pants on and my dress socks pulled up to my knees, so if you squint a little, I looked like a shorter version. He looked at me and took in all that glory, and then smiled. "You're going to be awesome, babe," which he has said to me a majillion times before in the span of our relationship.

Our wedding day? "You're awesome. Let's go."

First pregnancy? "It'll be awesome. Let's do this."

Scary C-section and all that mess? "So awesome. I'm proud of you."

My first big speaking gig was when *Bottled* came out, and I called him from backstage two minutes before the intro? "Babe. Remember why you're doing this. And you'll be awesome." He simply believed it. Incidentally, all those things ended up being awesome.

I stared at him. And then I put on some pants. I should just believe him. He's been right all those times before.

The real deal here is that Brian's faith in me simply reminded me of my faith in myself. He mirrored it right back my way.

And, afterward, according to Brian, my talk "Was awesome!"[14]

I was still nervous. When I was back in the green room and then backstage, I did deep breathing and a few power kicks to remind myself of my Super Woman status. I stood with my feet wide, hands on hips, and pictured my cape, fluttering behind me. "You got this," the sound girl whispered to me as she affixed the mic pack to my hip. "You're gonna rock it." I wanted to hug her, but there were cords involved now.

When I walked out to applause and the lights that blinded me, I took a deep breath and began. Brian and my friends were in the front row, or at least I think so. Because the lights were so intense, I wasn't really sure. But about twenty seconds in, I heard it. I had made the first significant point in my talk, and I heard it, a soft, sort of "Yes, girl" hum from the audience. I knew that sound. My friend Anita was "Mmm hmmmm"-ing to me.

Anita is a "Mmm-hmm-er." She does this when she sits next to me in church. She "mmm-hmms" when she's gathered with people and is listening along. That "mmm-hmm" is Anita's calling card. She's an outward listener, all leaning in and throaty humming to really let you know your words are being soaked up and fully appreciated by the therapist/friend/superwoman that is Anita. The first time I heard it during my TEDx talk, I almost broke my pace. "Hark!" my inner Dana shouted, "Is that an Anita I detect on yonder horizon?"

Yeah, I don't really know why my inner Dana is kind of Shakespearean, but zounds, it is what it is.

From thereon, I heard the gentle hmm-hmming of Anita at multiple points in my talk, and this spurred me on. Anita's verbal tic saved the day. Brian's unfettered optimism saved the day. Their support reminded me of who I was. And then I stood up and saved the day.

So I trusted the support system I had. I've been working with this support system for years; it has been built and fortified by good people and good wisdom.

But while I was working on this book, I realized there was another key element that strengthened me and helped me stand up that day. Patterns. And I do *love* a good pattern.

When I was around twelve, my dad took me to JCPenney to buy me a trench coat. I don't know why my dad wanted me to have a trench coat. The whole thing was just weird because Dad was not in charge of the shopping at our house. If my mom were with me, we would have hit the mall, maybe The Limited in the back where the sales racks were, and yet here we were, at JCPenney's, looking for a trench coat.

I did not want a trench coat. Nobody who is twelve wants a trench coat. My friend Heidi had a bright red woolen Gap coat with black toggle buttons. I wanted that coat. Instead, I got a brown trench coat that was a little too long for me and made me look like Inspector Gadget.

I have always wanted to ask my dad about the trench coat incident. Did he suddenly decide he wanted to help me with my fashion sense? Did he have a desire to turn his twelve-year-old daughter into Columbo? There was never another shopping expedition with Dad, for which I am grateful. I don't really know where that coat ended up. I never liked it.

But a couple of years ago, the trenchcoat episode was redeemed at a thrift store, on one of my endless searches for baskets. As I was walking down an aisle of jackets, I spotted something, a cream trench. I don't really know what drew me to it, except it looked to be in pristine condition, and I slowly pulled it out and eyed it. Maybe . . . maybe I could rock a trench now? I could cinch it tight around my waist and look cool, like Uma Thurman. And that's when I saw it. The inside lining peeked out, an iconic pattern of creamy camel, red, and black plaid. I gasped a little and looked around. Was this a Burberry coat? What in the world was a Burberry trench doing in our little thrift store in the Midwest? I grasped at the collar and there it was, *"Burberrys" Made in England,* carefully embroidered.

Yes, it could have been a fake. But I checked the buttons. I googled the tag. I kept coming up with confirmation. This was, most likely, the real deal. And it was *six dollars.*

So, I bought the coat. I think I texted Brian about my find, and he responded with his usual "That's great, honey!" with no actual idea what he was talking about.[15] When I tried it on at home, I looked like a short person trying to wear a trench coat, but still. I own a Burberry trench coat now, and occasionally I will bring it out if it's raining, or if I want to look like Inspector Gadget.

If you're sort of into fashion, even despite that you're a middle-aged mom in the Midwest, you can spot a Burberry plaid anywhere. It's a classic. Queen Elizabeth was often seen wearing their trench with a brown, red, and black Burberry scarf neatly tucked around her neck. She had granted the brand a Royal Warrant as "Official Weatherproofer" back in 1955. It's iconic stuff.

But in the past few years, Burberry has raised some traditionalists' eyebrows with a risky pattern evolution. Burberry's plaid can now be spotted on the runway in deep indigos, ruby reds, or bright mustards. The pattern was there, but so was playfulness and change.

This was my life. I took what I knew and built on the pattern. I have been constructing my own evolutions, stitching creativity and bravery together since I got sober.

Here's a timeline of my own pattern evolution:

2011: Original sobriety date. After three years, I relapsed for a week over the Christmas holiday. Nothing says the birth of Jesus like sneaking vodka out of a plastic bottle in your closet. It was awful and blessedly short.

2014: New Year's Day. New sobriety date.

2015: A publisher contacted me about an article I wrote about being a mom of toddlers while maintaining my sobriety. They asked me to write a book, and I wrote *Bottled: A Mom's Guide to Early Recovery.* It takes nine months and is my third child, and life-changing for me. I became a "real writer." This is something I have wanted since I was a little girl.

2018: I wrote *How to BePerfect Like Me*. This was about the relapse, and it was a lot tougher to create. It was raw and refining, and you know I struggled. But what doesn't kill us . . .

2019–2020: All sorts of weird stuff is going on. See Chapters 1–8. Not much writing. Miserable.

2021: On a whim, I decided to try stand-up comedy.

2022: I do stand-up again. Glutton for punishment and all that.

2022: After not doing much writing for over five years, I think, *You know. I think I'd like to try and write a book about aging and menopause, and my recovery. I hope someone might want to read it?*[16]

2023: I start writing again, regularly, for *Psychology Today* and other publications. Oh, and after months of trying, I finally secured an agent. Dani is my hero.

2024: I do a TEDx talk about my gray hair.

And here we are.

All of this was an organic unfolding of the original pattern: Keep creating. Keep writing. Evolve and flow.

When I performed stand-up the second time, Jeremy brought in a comedian from the Twin Cities, Ali Horman. Ali's been performing for over ten years. When Ali writes comedy, something very specific happens to her brain. The thinkie part, the prefrontal cortex, powers down. The prefrontal cortex wants to say, "You know, this should be funny. You should really try hard to be funny right now. THINK HARDER." This is unhelpful.

Instead, the temporal cortex steps up to the plate. This is the portion of the brain that gathers and syncs up language, visual memories, and emotions into a verdant, messy mass, taking things that look disparate and disconnected and linking them, like the florid wallpaper in our guest bath that is jumbled but still works somehow. Comedy is often about connecting the unexpected, and this portion of the brain is about gathering these different images, memories, and emotions, and making some sense of them. It's like when the art instructor steps away from the pedagogy and then just watches her students pick up their brushes and create, in lovely, maybe a little chaotic, freedom.

When I was teaching high school English, we sometimes journaled at the beginning of the hour, just to get the creative juices flowing. I gave them a prompt, like a song, and then I'd let them go for about ten minutes. Some would sit there, twiddling a pen between their fingers, stuck. I'd quote one of my favorite baseball movies, *Bull Durham*, where Kevin Costner admonishes his pitcher to stop overthinking his game. "Don't think," he'd say. "Don't think. Just *throw*."[17] I would scrawl that up on my whiteboard at the front of the room in large letters:

DON'T THINK. JUST THROW.

Working on a comedy show script was unlike any other writing assignment I had accomplished. It used totally different skills and strategies. It was also terrifying. All that stretching and surprise led me to write again.

After writer's block, feeling stuck, and afraid, I started again. I stood up for myself. I believed that I had something worthwhile to say. I took a deep breath, and I threw the ball.

Two (long) years later, I had a book deal.

One of the TEDx speakers had an adorable daughter who drew a picture of me during dress rehearsal. Perhaps this should be my new headshot (Figures 12.1 and 12.2).

Stand Up

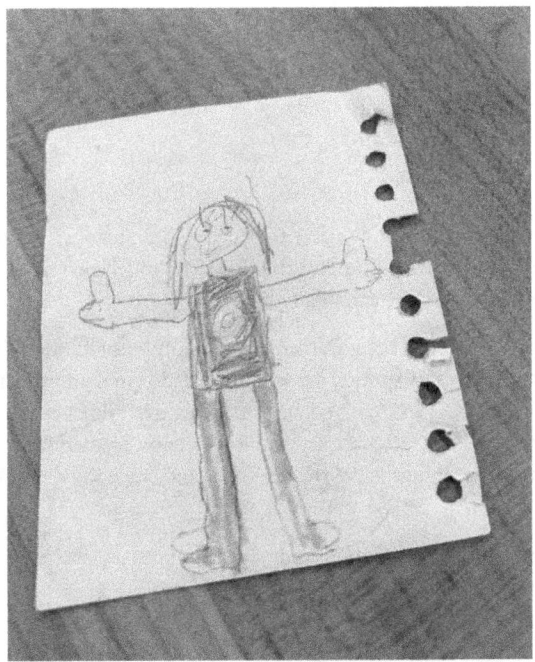

Figure 12.1 *Here I am in my fabulous pink suit pants and I guess a metal band t-shirt.*

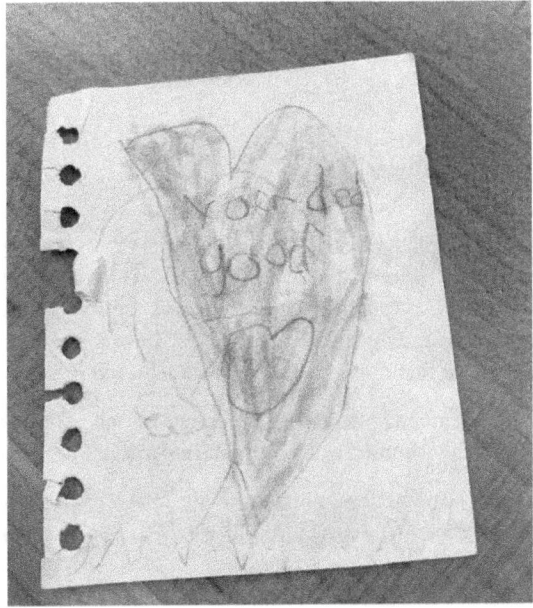

Figure 12.2 *"You ded good."*

Notes

1. Jaron has since gone on to have a really successful comedic career, and so I get to say I opened for him. In a backyard.

2. Comedians.

3. It's weird when you write it and realize that saying Yes meant *stopping* something. Usually, it's the other way around. But this wasn't so much saying Yes and stopping. It was more like saying Yes and starting to listen to myself.

4. Shameless plug for my first book *Bottled* that goes into much more detail here, but let's just say that Brian was spotted across a crowded room, and the magical seas parted, and lo, he was The ONE. Whatever that means. I don't even know what that means. But I really "knew" (with finger quotes) when I spotted him. He was wearing a Hawaiian shirt and standing over by the food, and since then, that has pretty much not changed.

5. The movie *Yes Day*, starring Garner and a bunch of other people, was way cute, but it did raise my kids' expectations a bit too high.

6. Kittens were up for negotiation.

7. This is not true. They are fed and watered daily.

8. Try it! Stop reading! Do it right now! It's miraculous.

9. Dad's nickname has been The Silver Fox for as long as I can remember. He has a real Cary Grant kind of thing going on.

10. That's fifty. They don't even like to say the number. It's the Age-That-Must-Not-Be-Named.

11. I still do.

12. MHUTOASPUYGRVYLELUSUPPSUP.

13. One bag was entirely devoted to cords for devices. The mammoth size of that bag is directly related to the probability that he will not have the right connector for things. He also has a box in his office that I have labeled "Cords for things we don't own anymore," but I know. I know he's waiting. There will come a day when he will be able to go through that box, and one of those suckers will work, and he will lift it to the heavens in triumph. At that moment, he will have achieved Peak Male.

14. Honestly, I don't remember. I often don't remember my talks. I know I heard a few women shouting "Whoo-hoos!!" as I left the stage. So, that's awesome enough for me.

15. Sixty-five percent of our marriage is just us saying "That's great, honey!" with no actual clue what the other person is talking about. This works very well.

16. THANK YOU!

17. Brian! Lookit! A sports analogy!

Bibliography

1. **On a daily basis, humans say yes six times more to others than they say no:**
Price, Jenna (2023, April 19). Humans Ask for Help Every Couple of Minutes, and We Mainly Say Yes. *Brisbane Times*. https://tinyurl.com/86seukwv.

2. **Did you know that a straight posture helps us remember good memories more often than bad ones?**
Peper, Erik, I-Mei Lin, Richard Harvey, and Jacob Perez (2017, April). How Posture Affects Memory Recall and Mood. *ResearchGate*. Association for Applied Psychophysiology and Biofeedback. https://www.researchgate.net/publication/321348063_How_Posture_Affects_Memory_Recall_and_Mood.

3. **...a part of my brain can threaten to shut down:**
Sewell, Helen (2016, February 25). Public Speaking Anxiety Shuts down the Brain. *Simply Speaking*. https://tinyurl.com/rzm4y6e4.

4. **Invisible Women Syndrome is a researched phenomenon:**
Gransnet (2016). Invisibility in Later Life Survey Results. https://www.gransnet.com/online-surveys-product-tests/feeling-invisible-survey-data-results.

5. **We're left out of clinical trials and medical research, both for our gender:**
Blakemore, Erin (2022, June 27). Women Are Still Underrepresented in Clinical Trials. *Washington Post*. https://www.washingtonpost.com/health/2022/06/27/underrepresentation-women-clinical-trials/.

6. **...and our age:**
Goodwin, Victoria A., Margaret Low, Terence J. Quinn, Emma Cockcroft, Victoria Shepherd, Philip Evans, Emily Henderson, et al. (2023). Including Older People in Health and Social Care Research: Best Practice Recommendations Based on the INCLUDE Framework. *Age and Ageing* 52 (6). https://doi.org/10.1093/ageing/afad082.

7. **...yet the physical and mental ramifications of menopause are still underresearched:**
NIH MedlinePlus Magazine (2023, September 12). What We Know—and Still Don't Know—about Menopause. https://magazine.medlineplus.gov/article/what-we-know-and-still-dont-know-about-menopause.

8. **People fear public speaking more than death:**
Brewer, Geoffrey (2001, March 19). Public Speaking Anxiety. *National Social Anxiety Center*. https://nationalsocialanxietycenter.com/social-anxiety/public-speaking-anxiety/#:~:text=The%20fear%20of%20public%20speaking.

9. **She had granted the brand a Royal Warrant as "Official Weatherproofer" back in 1955:**
Burberry (2022). Our History. https://us.burberry.com/c/our-history/.

10. **When Ali writes comedy something very specific happens to her brain:**
Byrne, Dom (2023, March). What Happens in Our Brains When We're Trying to Be Funny. *Nature*. https://doi.org/10.1038/d41586-023-00627-8.

13

Forgiveness and Permission

*Forgiveness liberates the soul, it removes fear. That's
why it's such a powerful weapon.*
NELSON MANDELA

This is the chapter where I have to apologize to the UPS lady because I was a jerk. It's also the chapter where I analyze words like "forgiveness," "grace," and "nutball" within an inch of their lives.

Process addictions don't just get obliterated by really healthy, disciplined, "Day One" behavior. They're too sneaky for that. They play whack-a-mole with my brain, and the only way to work it out is to start permitting myself to fail. Daily. This is tough. Drinking is a big fat NO, so shouldn't I keep that total abstinence mindset with donuts? How do I navigate this?

With forgiveness and permission.

To begin, let's cover some rules. Forgiveness does not cover a tricky little thing called the non-apology. Non-apologies usually start with something like "Well, I'm sorry if . . . " or even worse, "I'm sorry. But . . . " Both of these are sorry frauds. Non-apologies like to play a shell game that ends in defeat. I can watch the shell, peer at it with intensity and even confidence, but when it's all over the only thing I'm left with is emptiness. And, perhaps a little rage.

My husband and I played this game early in our marriage. We hadn't learned how to take our time with each other when we were angry. "I'm sorry, but I just don't understand how you are ALWAYS late," I would say, after trying to keep his dinner from congealing. In my first year of marriage, I took great pains to make all the dinners or help Brian pack for a work trip, or even, Lord help me, iron his clothes. These were tasks that would prove (to me) that I was the Perfect Wife, something I was very interested in back then. About a year in, I was super stressed and had a lot of hidden resentments. But I kept this up, and then I would drink about four glasses of wine while I, the domestic goddess, prepared a lovely meal, only to watch the meal attach itself to the pan in a sodden mess because Brian worked late again.

Yes, he was wrong; he should have called. He was also a workaholic, a perfectionist, and a slew of other bad things that I was able to judge him for, while at the same time, I was exhibiting the same behaviors. This is marriage.

Thus, we would argue, and I would be shrill, and then I would stomp upstairs and go to bed mad, and we would repeat this about two times a week. He would apologize the next morning, and I would too, but I would do the "I'm sorry but" kind, so it didn't count. He would lob this kind of apology back at me as well. "I'm sorry I was grumpy. But I just can't seem to understand why you can't SHUT anything. Our air conditioning bill is astronomical," and I stopped listening after "I just can't" because it was a sham. This brand of apology means nothing.

It's the first year of marriage. What are you gonna do? That first year is when you start to notice that he never hangs up a washcloth. He wads it up in the corner of the shower because he's a monster, and then you go and have a boring argument about a washcloth. During the washcloth argument, you pile on a few other things like a lost dental bill, that he drives too fast, and slowly, your marital bliss gets stuck under a pile of clutter in his office that he never deals with.

Marriage is fun that way.

So, those are the apologies that don't count at all. Just to be clear. Just to establish some rules.

Because rules are needed when talking about something like forgiveness. It's tricky.

Where do I start? I could go over the wreckage of my past. I could list for you the horrible things I did when I was drinking and how those moments like to surface now, like dead fish in a pond for me to shudder at when it's 3:20 in the morning. I could do that.

I could tell you how I try to stop these memories and say a prayer for them, and act "as if." I say out loud, "That's forgiven, Dana," because I still need the reminder. I still need to hear it out loud.

Or I could tell you about how I still have resentments, like with my husband, for example, and they need to be dealt with. Forgiven. I have a whole pack of resentments shoved in my back pocket that, if I reach for just one, all of them can come fluttering out. These resentments are about his lousy behavior, but they inevitably make *me* the one with the lousy behavior, and this is just so unfair. There is forgiveness needed here too, in a thick application, on both sides now.

But wait, there's more. Beyond spouses, there are parents. That's a biggie. We have to forgive the parents; they're a mess too. We parents botch it up, like *all* the time. Honestly, it's embarrassing. Oh, and friends? Sometimes friends can be awful. It's so weird how people just keep blowing it. Why do they do that?

While I'm at it, I would also like to share that when Brian and I were planning our wedding, I asked my then-pastor to marry us, and he had to decline. He said he was traveling, I think? I was disappointed because I loved this guy. He was personable and warm, and I felt like he'd had such a large part in establishing my faith. I'd only been attending church for about six years when I started attending his church, and I loved it there. It was home.

A year later, I found out that he'd been having an affair with the church music director for years. So, as I sat in my pew and listened to him talk about being authentic and seeking truth, and I nodded along, he was a liar. So, I have to forgive him, too, I guess?

Oh, and I'm still mad about Bill Cosby. He was my comedy hero and America's Dad. My sister Jenni and I would put his album *I Started Out as a Child* on the record player, and we'd laugh so hard our stomachs would hurt. We could quote the entire thing. This was our childhood, and he's just awful, and he took that from me, those memories with my sister. I need to forgive him for messing up what a hero is.

I guess I should also forgive politicians and presidents who ask for fidelity and want us to wave flags and believe and hope, and then they act like scumbags.

It's a lot.

I'm tired.

So, I guess I could start with something small. Me?

But I'm not feeling all that small. Here's why. I had a full day all to myself. Nothing on the calendar. No kids. The house was still and tidy, and I was going to spend the entire day in wonderful industrious creativity: writing, planning, and ten hours of focused dedication to the writerly life. I woke up with a deep sense of gratitude for these plans. It was one I had always dreamed of, writing the day away with an actual book deadline. I had my supplies all set up in the living room, where the light was creamy and lovely in the early morning: my computer, my standing desk, a fresh stack of notebooks, and colored pens. The whole thing had a tang of industriousness and optimism.

And I blew it. I completely blew it.

After I dropped the boys off at school, I started out strong. I went for a run. I climbed the stairs and started to make our bed. "Just a quick tidy up. But I'll sit down by 9:30," I told our cats Lucy and Milk. They followed me to the bathroom as I took my shower, and then I got sidetracked with some laundry. I made it to my seat around 10 a.m. No biggie. No problem. So far, so good. And then I tried to write something. I looked at my notes. I started to research octopus moms. I checked my emails. I tried to write again.

Each sentence felt sticky like it needed to be scraped off the bottom of my brain. This was uncomfortable. And there was a rude buzzing behind my eyes, right in the center of my forehead. I wrote six sentences.

Is it a headache? Or is it depression?

So yeah. That all started up at 10:30. I got up and made a fresh batch of coffee. The stove was filthy. I scratched at some baked-on pasta with my fingernail.

I decided that I should go play fetch with Pepper, our tank/German Shepherd puppy. Her love language is "clobber." This should help.

I played fetch with the linebacker in the backyard. I hydrated properly. I tried to work out the chapter in my head, but what I kept thinking was that nobody on *Virgin River* ever tells the other characters what is going *on*. They're not even keeping secrets, per se. The characters just leave out glaringly important information constantly with each other, like they all have some sort of amnesia. Then they look conflicted and say they have to go get lunch, and they leave. People would be so much happier on that show if they just got into the details. So, I rewrite season five for them in my head. Also, how do the Virgin River people get away with constantly dining out at the one restaurant in town? That has to be so *expensive*.

I sit down again. Pepper is excited and wipes her face on me. I get up to wipe off dog snot. Rey, our other dog, looks sad. I go to cuddle her because she feels very left out since Pepper is here. She's devastated. I lie on the couch with her and try to think like a dog. It doesn't get either of us anywhere.

I'm on the couch now, though. With a dog.

Couch = food. It's Pavlovian, which is fitting because there's a dog here. My stomach rumbles faintly. Also? Writing is boring sometimes. It's just me, me, me, which is usually my thing, but there's that added step of typing.

Maybe I need a bit of a break from all this writing I have been doing. Also, there are apple fritters in the kitchen. I could start on season 6 of *Virgin River*. But just for a little bit. Just one episode. Just one fritter. Rey waits for me to come back with my fritters and my excuses, and she sighs contentedly as I settle in. I am helping her mental state, so this is worth it.

I eat too much sugar. The buzzing behind my eyes increases. *Virgin River* seems to help. I pull a blanket over Rey and me, and I don't move for another two hours.

But that's just a break! I can still fix this. I can still make the afternoon all about writing and productivity! I can turn this neurotic Titanic around! There's still time!

I don't move. A body wedged on a couch stays on a couch. It's science. I vow to get up tomorrow at 5 a.m. to make up for it. I needed this time off, right? I guess I also needed about a solid pound of carbs too. The boys come home and ask where the fritters are. I feel shaky and tired.

So . . . "starting small" is not accurate. I feel bloated and huge, a big ol' lump of fail.

And shame lurches around in my mind too. It had started as a small chunk, around 9 a.m., but by the end of the day, it was all bloated too.

Shame doesn't understand apologies. It's too primeval for that. It communicates in grunts and by thwacking me with things and making incoherent demands. And shame is big and sticky, and it makes me feel afraid, but also kind of grossed out.

Shame is Jabba the Hutt. (And there. Right there, I have established my nerd status.)

Shame makes it hard. And life is hard enough. I remember long ago when the boys were toddlers, I related a particularly shaming parenting moment to my friend Beth. "I just kind of snapped," I said to her. Both boys had decided to festoon the playroom with Hi Ho Cherry-O! pieces because flinging tiny red cherries all over the place was way more fun than playing a game with them. I'd had a tough day, or at least I used that as my excuse, but what did I know? It had probably been a day like all the others. My boys were still little and cute and said things like "Yes Mama" when I asked them things.

But I yelled at them. "WHY?" I yelled. "WHY would you do this?" Neither of them came through in this moment. They just sat there, and Steve the cat sauntered in and lay down on a pile of pieces because he always did that when people were mad. He liked to diffuse the situation. He eyed me with a slow blink. "Lay off the boys," he seemed to say. "They'll clean it up and I'll watch."

I didn't lay off. I yelled some more. Then I started in on a lecture about how I had just CLEANED that room and now we had to CLEAN it all AGAIN, and if a mom says this speech in a playroom, and two toddlers aren't really listening, did the speech happen at all?

Beth listens in the mom version, which means she is also wiping down a child or putting something back. But she listens.

And I slump against the wall in the playroom and admit to Beth the Big Kahuna: my greatest fear. "I mean. Is this all there is? Just this endless screwing up? I can handle it when it's just me messing up with me, but now there are others" I nod in the direction of my sons. "There are OTHER people who are attached to my mess-ups. They're going down with me. And Beth, it won't stop. I'll just keep doing it to them. It's unforgivable."

Beth wiped down another kid and said, "But that's the deal. All moms do this. And that's life. This is what it's like to be a parent. And if not," she smiles wickedly, "We would miss out on ALL this." She gestures widely at one kid who walks by with a sagging diaper. The air is fragrant. He has drool festooning his face and is gnawing on a slimy toy, and I'm sure there are some more bodily fluids packed into this moment. I laugh weakly.

She took her child to hose him down, and I started cleaning up while telling my toddlers to do it. We sang the cleanup song. It was a metaphor.

Beth and I both worked outside of the home full-time, so this conversation had to be on a Saturday morning. I took the boys to the house, and then I cleaned and cooked, and meal prepped for the week because that's what working as a mom meant. Three jobs for the price of one. I didn't seem to question it back then; I just did these things, probably because relinquishing control of my mom and wife duties would mean failure. Later, when the boys were older, I finally had a total meltdown and didn't clean the house for over a week until someone noticed that things were piling up in weird places. Brian and I had a discussion. He said, "How can I help?" I blinked and realized that I was enraged, which was too bad for Brian, as he thought he was being nice. I said, "I don't want you to *help*. I want you to DO." He told me to write down a list. Make a list of the things I needed him to do. I told him I didn't want to make a list.

Actually, I yelled. Yes, there was yelling. But I don't remember feeling all that bad about it.

It worked itself out. We have a better rhythm now, but I still end up cleaning all the things, and that's on me. I can't help it. Anyone who has ever rage-cleaned the kitchen knows: It's therapy and it's anti-bacterial. Incidentally, Brian is still a slob, and I still get mad about it. We are just more aware of the process. He leaves a bike helmet, two wrenches, and his athletic cup on the dining room table, and then he says, "I know that's there. I will move it later today." He doesn't move it for two weeks, and I end up praying about my anger over an athletic cup. As is the way. We move in and out of daily forgiveness because we've been married forever, and we have outside help.

If you don't believe in God, then more power to you. Literally. I have to believe because I can't do any of this on my own. When I got sober, that was one of the first rules: let go and let God. And it's also the only way I can do forgiveness. I'd been a Christian since I was twenty-eight. I found Jesus, which always makes him sound like he was stuffed under the couch cushions, and I found a new peace. But I also compartmentalized Jesus, which is tough since he's everywhere. I told him I was for him except for this "one thing." The drinking. The drinking was still mine, and that bargaining went on for another twelve years.

The thing with faith is that it comes off as crazy.

Also, religion can get messed up. Have you noticed? Church betrayals hurt. And then there's the patriarchy, hypocrisy, and lies. It's a whole thing.

But see, I have this little church. It's where I spend Sunday mornings. It's full of messed-up people who are the kindest and most generous folks I know. It's peaceful there. Well, sometimes it's not because Darrel and Jeff specialize in sermons that perform surgery, and that can be a lot. But the music helps. We have a banjo player. I ask a lot of questions there, and the pastors put up with that. Sometimes I cry. I stare straight ahead and try not to wipe my face because I don't want anyone to notice. Inevitably, I get too damp and usually Henry notices because he's a noticer of these things. He'll smile at me because he's used to me. I'm a church-crier. I'll lean over and whisper, "Get me a tissue, like seventeen of them," and he'll hop up, happy to get out of the sermon for a bit.

I talk to God every day, even when I'm cussing, and I often ask him to help me find my car keys, which is dumb because he's busy. I rail at him about pain and the awful world. I repeatedly ask Jesus to explain stuff I don't understand. I ask even louder for him to explain the lousy stuff I do. I wonder if he gets tired of it. I also thank him a lot, and I mix him up in my mind with the Jesus actor from *The Chosen* and warn him I might get confused when I die and meet him, and he doesn't look like Jonathan Roumie. "I get that a lot," Jesus says. "But, I'm better looking if you can believe it."

I believe. Help me in my unbelief.

I cart around unbelief.

That cart gets a little lighter when I go to recovery meetings because that is where I meet up with God. When I got sober, my life became about just breathing in and out and not dying and not drinking. Maybe there are no alcoholic atheists in foxholes. I needed faith. I had to have it. I drank it up when I got sober, and I am still so sure of it—as I am sure that sitting here writing these words might alienate or frustrate or turn some of you off. But, I am just sure of God.

Until I'm not. And then we talk. It's complicated.

Since the late 1990s, research on spirituality and health has rapidly increased. There is a connection between improved mental health and spirituality. Hope was quantified in these studies. Hope was... *healthy*. Faith can be a determining factor that reduces cravings. In one study, participants who were in long-term recovery were scanned via an MRI while being shown images of drinks. Then, each participant was either given some neutral reading material or was asked to read and recite the serenity prayer. The serenity prayer group reported fewer cravings after the prayer, and follow-up MRIs coincided. The prefrontal cortex responded differently. Portions of the brain in charge of emotional processing responded differently. It was like the prayer-brain was just more agile and prepared to deal with the triggers and the want of alcoholism than the non-prayer one.

Wanting was what hurt me when I was trying to get sober. And it's the wanting that still trips me up. It's not for alcohol, not a craving for a cold glass of wine. Those images I see on the television (because people drink constantly on TV) with the reward of pouring a glass of wine because it has become a personality trait for their (always female) characters; they don't make me want wine.

Instead, I want forgiveness. It's about forgiving myself. Still.

Here's a recent and really fun conversation we had at our house:

TV: We interrupt the Royals game with a commercial about this supercool new alcoholic beverage that markets itself as containing "real juice" and is in a pink and yellow can that is cute and kidlike.

Me: So, next juice boxes. Basically, they are going to start marketing alcoholic juice boxes.

Teenage child: Have you seen Twisted Tea? It looks just like an energy drink.

Me: *Narrows eyes and focuses on the kid. You can hear my Alcoholic Mom in Recovery Spidey Sense start tingling.*

Teenage child: What? Why does your face look like that?

Me: Have YOU "seen" Twisted Tea? How do you know about these alcohol things? When was this a point of discussion? Where? Why?

Teenage child: What? What is happening?

Me: TELL ME THE TRUTH.

Teenage child: MOM. I CAN DO ALL CAPS TOO.

Me: FIFTY PERCENT OF-

Teenage child: I'm going upstairs to stare at my phone.

It's so hard. It's his life, but don't you see? I might have destroyed it. But it's still his life to destroy. And when I use words like "destroy," he says that's "dramatic" and I need to "calm down," and honestly, I probably do. These conversations are periodic and increasingly capable of freaking me out. What if I have ruined him? How can I forgive myself for that?

Also, there's this:

Me: Well, it's been a stressful day.

Couch, the cast of *Virgin River*, and apple fritters: We know what to do.

And finally, this:

Me: *Looks around house in various states of mess* I'm tired.

Husband: How about you go rest? Put your feet up! Take a nap.

Husband: But also, in about four minutes? I'm going to wake you up and ask you where the spatula is.

Rage: I'm on it.

It's my continued messing up that begs for forgiveness. And I hate it. I don't even know how to forgive others very well at all, and I have no idea how to get started on myself. I get stuck in this no-man's land:

Forgiving others =

Oops! Page cannot load! Log in first under Application to Self

Forgiving self =

Oops! Password not recognized! Log in first under Application to Others

Did you know? "Self-forgiveness" is never mentioned in the bible. I found this confusing, and when I asked my pastor about it, he answered, "That's because it's not even really a thing. It's not a theological issue at all. It's not possible."

I love talking to Darrell. He's the one at the party who will come up to you and ask, "Now, how are you, really?" when everyone else is talking about how Kathy brought homemade ice cream for the party. And he'll stand there and wait while you answer, even while that ice cream is rapidly disappearing, because he wants to know, right then, that you might be struggling with writing a chapter about forgiveness. Part of you realizes that now you're in the thick of it, and there's no going back. Your husband brings you ice cream, and Darrel tries to explain.

But he doesn't lead well. "Yeah. Forgiveness is really hard. Like, *really* hard. But the self-forgiveness stuff . . . " he takes a pause. "I just don't believe it's possible without God."

This is a big statement, but he's a pastor, so he can do stuff like that.

As he talks, I start to relax. I understand what he's saying. Self-forgiveness isn't a part of biblical theology because it's illusory. We don't need it because we already have it. It's already a done deal. All my agonizing and fear and pain—those feelings might be real, but they are all just a conversation I have that is also outside of my control. The relief is palpable.

I believe. Help me in my unbelief.

Forgiveness is faith, as a breath of prayer, that gives me a deep gust of wind to set my sails alight. To keep me upright and moving.

It's a bit woo-woo, if you ask me. It asks a lot, and it asks nothing. At the same time.

My first impression of faith, when I was twenty-eight and desperate enough to contemplate ending my existence on this planet, was that I had nothing to give anymore. I was just a big hole of emptiness. There was no way I was going to be able to fix the situation in my own time or with my own brain, like ever. So, I just lay in my bed one night and asked the ceiling: "I have no idea if you even exist. I don't. But if you do, you need to show up right now or I'm going to head out."

I was so tired. I was just so tired of relying on myself all the time.

And God did show up. The only way I can describe it is a feeling of relief. A lightness. A deep understanding that I was loved.

It's a big woo-woo again. But it happened.

God came through. He said, "I got you. Let's get to work. Oh, and in about ten years your life is gonna blow up, but let's just start here, shall we?"

And so we did. I was hunched over in a puddle of defeat back then. I was exhausted from grief. Jesus carted me around most of the time.

And it's THAT brand of lumpiness that takes me right up to trying to forgive myself for the wreckage of addiction. When I try to comprehend the colossal awfulness that is addiction, family, and stakes, I become a blob of worry and fatigue.

I forgive. Help me in my unforgiveness.

And here is the astonishing part. I accept being a lump in this case. This is not couch-lumping! This is something completely different! It's a sagging heap of healing and weirdness! I can finally relax!

Pfft, you say. *It's just a mind game, Dana. It's a trick. And we know that tricks are traps. They aren't real.*

If I chose to forgive someone, it might be a muttering of a sort of wishy-washy prayer or a half-assed "I forgive you" like when I used to make my sons say "I'm sorry" in that scripted way that moms make their kids do. Ineffectual? Maybe. Cute? Yes. Anyhow, it might seem like there's nothing really happening with all these "sorrys," but the brain is actually responding. Forgiveness, in speech or feeling, activates the portion of the brain where empathy and sympathy emotions reside. It helps with depression and anxiety. Forgiveness boosts the immune system. It can even reduce the risk of a heart attack. And, in my case, most interestingly, people with substance abuse disorders who practice forgiveness have a lower risk of relapsing.

So forgiveness is awesome! It's a health plan! It should go on the road! Why aren't more people signing up?

Because it's freaking hard, that's why. It's basically praying, which is not always my favorite thing. Too many unknowns.

Forgiveness is hard because people hurt us. I once had a friend who did a schmuck thing, and it was awful. No, I'm not going to go into the details because that would be uncool, but let's describe, as vaguely as possible, how hurt can just sit in your soul until you want to puke. She was my friend. I trusted her. She was also in recovery, so that made us even tighter. This person never gave me any red flags. Our relationship was healthy, wonderful, and solid. So, after a lot of thought, I worked up the courage to tentatively ask for a writing favor from her. She had the connections, and she enthusiastically agreed. She was a huge fan of my writing! My relief was palpable.

And then, she disappeared. No, not literally. She's still around. Still happily living her life, posting on social media about her world, still sober, I think. But as for me? She ghosted me so hard that I hear a scary soundtrack whenever I think about her.

I reached out—emails, messages, even phone calls (I know, right? Talk about a scary movie). She never responded. I racked my brain because it had to be me. I had to have done something horrible. I pored over memories and yes, even my books, to make sure I had not said something, done something. I would lie awake at night, willing the ceiling to tell me: WHAT DID I DO?

I wasn't done. I started polling my friends. I mean, I *have* friends. (I kept muttering this to myself.) I have friends, so I don't think it's because I was a horrible friend to her. I texted my friends. I asked my husband, "Am I a good person?" to which he responded without a breath, "Indubitably." No one ever says "indubitably" anymore, so I bought it. I would find myself staring into space about once a day, shocked into remembering: Oh, wait. I have someone who completely left me, and I should ruminate on that right now to try and figure it out. This is tough when I'm trying to do other things too, like write. Writing just begs for any sort of diversion because it feels like taking the brain on a long run with hills, so trying to figure out the ghosting thing? A wonderful distraction. Also, completely traumatizing, because I must be a horrible writer, and that's why this is happening, but I was willing to go there every day.

For weeks, I lived like this. My rumination and I were besties. My hurt sat in my chest. I had to figure this out.

And then, one afternoon, as I had yet again swerved into the weeds of paranoid sleuthing and people-solving, I remembered something.

It was an old faith-y trick that my mom had taught me long ago, about prayer. I didn't do anything with it for ages because I didn't want to be a faith-y person. They were weird. But I figured I was weird enough now, so I'd give it a shot.

"The thing with forgiveness, Dana," she said, "is it's not a feeling. You just do it." I sighed. This was just the kind of theological instruction that made me twitch. It followed along with my recovery group's firm adherence to the other nutball "acting as if" thing, which I know works, but still. Just forgiving people, all willy-nilly with no real hunkering down and trying to FEEL forgive-y was too vague. There were no parameters. It had no specifics. It was slippery, like the golden rule that people throw around, but that can be remodeled to fit any vibe. "Treat others as you want to be treated, Dana" someone spiritual intones, and I jut my chin and think, "Well I'm ok with being treated like a schmuck right now if I can turn it around and zap you with some of the same awfulness. That works for me just fine."

But then Mom said something about forgiveness that made me pay attention: "Just, pray for them. And not in a 'Lord, fix this awful person' way. Pray for them to be blessed. Like, a lot. Pray for God to just bless them a bunch and see what happens."

I guess I could do this. I mean, I could do it badly, but at least it was an action. I would slump into a posture of sulky prayer and I would say something like, "God, could you bless so and so today. Just make her have a blessed day because she's a loser and she needs it and blah blah blah bless bless bless," and I'd sort of mentally tick that off my list. And what would happen, like this was some sort of mystical Ready Bake Oven of goodness, was that within minutes I would *be less mad*. What I also noticed is that these target attacks of Blessing You Because I'm Mad At You prayers became stronger. They became more focused and thoughtful, less sulky. It took practice, but lo, it worked.

Forgiveness isn't a static personality trait. It can be practiced. It can be *learned*.

So that's what I did with this person. I took time and I prayed for her to get whacked over the head with all the wonderfulness that she could get in one day. I don't know if she's a Christian, but I dialed up Jesus so hard on her that I bet even if she didn't believe, she started having weird dreams about a guy that looked like Jonathan Roumie. But, I don't know. I still haven't heard from her, but I don't care anymore. I wish her well.

Also, just for your information, if she did contact me and wanted to explain? I am not sure I would take the call. I might. I don't know. Boundaries are just as valid as forgiveness. In fact, boundaries and forgiveness are best friends.

Both prayer and forgiveness look remarkably similar in how they function in my body. Just like forgiveness, prayer increases blood flow to the frontal lobes of the brain. Participating in prayer reduces stress in the body. It also benefits the immune system. It activates positive emotions and mental health. Prayer helps those in recovery to deal with cravings and stay sober. All of these attributes are the same markers for forgiveness.

So, maybe . . . Let's just see if I can work this out here. Maybe . . . I should try to forgive *myself* in the same way that I prayed blessings on those who hurt me?

Mind. Blown.

They build on each other: prayer and forgiveness. Interlocking into a repeated pattern to form a completed whole.

A Swedish mathematician, Helge von Koch, found that snowflakes follow a fractal pattern: one part of the snowflake, based on a simple triangle, repeats itself into infinity. If allowed to grow without melting, this fractal design would repeat itself until it was the size of the earth. That is one very special snowflake. Fractal patterns exist everywhere. It's why blood vessels look like streams. Or branches look like trees. It's a repeated progression of similar things making a whole, beautiful design.

It's why one day, when I was dropping off packages at the out-of-town UPS store, and I was told that I couldn't do so because I didn't have the right mailing labels for them. Then, I was a jerk about it, and I knew I had to say sorry. "It would have been nice to CLARIFY that on your website," I huffed. UPS was wrong. I had driven all the way here. I was tired. I was a jerk, and I made sure the clerk knew that my jerkiness was justified.

Pro tip: Jerk behavior is never justified.

Driving back home, I got quiet. I kept thinking about the conversation. But I wasn't thinking about it in the usual cacophony of how right I had been and how wrong UPS was. Instead, it was a simple pattern that I kept circling:

I messed up.

I needed to say sorry.

I finally took an exit and circled back, parked, and walked into the store. The girl eyed me, her face blank, waiting for the Karen to approach.

I walked up to her. "I didn't treat you at all well. It was my fault. You didn't deserve any of that. I am really sorry."

She blinked. And then she smiled. I smiled. She said, "Oh, that's ok, I've had way worse," which made me sad. And then, as I drove home to deal with packing labels another day, I felt so light and airy and, dare I say, happy, that I had to ruin it by trying to figure it out.

I think it's because by saying "sorry," out loud, I was able to be brave, to do something new, something that was outward, and then something that was inward. One thing looked like another thing. Forgiveness and faith. The pattern builds. And the parts heal into a whole.

How to forgive yourself in five easy steps:

1. Just kidding; it's not like that.
2. I like to remind myself that shame is a parasite. It attaches to all of this, and shame gloms up clear thinking. A good reset is to get outside.
3. I say, "I forgive you, Dana." I don't try to figure it out.
4. I put my hand on my belly. I breathe in love, and I breathe out pain.
5. I list three blessings in my life. There are so many of them; three is easy. It shifts something inside me, and it helps me remember: Do unto yourself as you would do unto others.
6. I repeat this often because if I don't, I forget the whole point. We all fail, and we must keep going. We simply must.

Bibliography

1 **Since the late 1990s, research on spirituality and health has rapidly increased:**
Koenig, Harold G. (2019). Religion, Spirituality, and Health: The Research and Clinical Implications. *ISRN Psychiatry* 2012 (278730): 1–33. https://doi.org/10.5402/2012/278730.

2 **Faith can be a determining factor that reduces cravings:**
Grim, Brian J., and Melissa E. Grim (2019). Belief, Behavior, and Belonging: How Faith is Indispensable in Preventing and Recovering from Substance Abuse. *Journal of Religion and Health* 58 (5): 1713–50. https://link.springer.com/article/10.1007/s10943-019-00876-w.

3 **Forgiving, in speech or feeling, activates the portion of the brain where empathy and sympathy emotions reside:**
Moawad, Heidi (2018, September 25). The Neurobiology of Forgiveness. *Neurology Live*. https://www.neurologylive.com/view/neurobiology-forgiveness.

4 **It helps with depression and anxiety:**
Templeton World Charity Foundation, Inc. (2023, April 20). "Largest-Ever Study on Forgiveness Shows Decreased Anxiety And . . .. https://www.templetonworldcharity.org/blog/REACH-forgiveness-study.

5 **Forgiveness boosts the immune system:**
Toussaint, Loren, Andrew J. Gall, Alyssa Cheadle, and David R. Williams (2019). Let It Rest: Sleep and Health as Positive Correlates of Forgiveness of Others and Self-Forgiveness. *Psychology & Health* 35 (3): 1–16. https://doi.org/10.1080/08870446.2019.1644335.

6 **It can even reduce the risk of heart attack:**
Hopkinsmedicine.org. (2021, November). Forgiveness: Your Health Depends on It. https://www.hopkinsmedicine.org/health/wellness-and-prevention/forgiveness-your-health-depends-on it#:~:text=The%20good%20news:%20Studies%20have.

7 **... people with substance abuse disorders who practice forgiveness have a lower risk of relapsing:**
Scherer, Michael, Everett L. Worthington, Joshua N. Hook, and Kathryn L. Campana (2011). "Forgiveness and the Bottle: Promoting Self-Forgiveness in Individuals Who Abuse Alcohol. *Journal of Addictive Diseases* 30 (4): 382–95. https://doi.org/10.1080/10550887.2011.609804.

8 **Forgiveness isn't a static personality trait. It can be practiced. It can be *learned*:**
Toussaint, Loren L., Grant S. Shields, and George M. Slavich (2016). Forgiveness, Stress, and Health: A 5-Week Dynamic Parallel Process Study. *Annals of Behavioral Medicine* 50 (5): 727–35. https://doi.org/10.1007/s12160-016-9796-6.

9 **Just like forgiveness, prayer increases blood flow to the frontal lobes of the brain:**
Elliott, Trisha (2015, January 30). New Research Says Praying Can Change Your Brain, No Kidding. *Broadview Magazine*. https://broadview.org/prayer-brain-research/#:~:text=Newberg%20reports%20increased%20activity%20in.

10 **Participating in prayer reduces stress in the body:**
Upenieks, Laura (2022). Unpacking the Relationship between Prayer and Anxiety: A Consideration of Prayer Types and Expectations in the United States. *Journal of Religion and Health* 62 (3): 1–22. https://doi.org/10.1007/s10943-022-01708-0.

11 **Prayer helps those in recovery to deal with cravings and stay sober:**
Greg, Williams (2016, May 3). Brain Images Reveal First Physical Evidence That Prayers Reduce Cravings in Alcoholics Anonymous Members. *NYU Langone News*. https://nyulangone.org/news/brain-images-reveal-first-physical-evidence-prayers-reduce-cravings-alcoholics-anonymous-members.

12 **A Swedish mathmetician, Helge von Koch, found that snowflakes follow a fractal pattern:**
GeeksforGeeks (2017, September 24). Koch Curve or Koch Snowflake. https://www.geeksforgeeks.org/koch-curve-koch-snowflake/.

13 **Fractals patterns exist everywhere:**
Barnett, Phil (2023, September 23). Why Do Things Look Like Other Things? *Microcosmic*. https://www.microcosmic.info/2017/09/why-do-things-look-like-other-things.html.

14

Foreverness

About a year before I got sober, I knew I was doomed. I had repeatedly tried to reel in my drinking. I scrabbled for rules that helped me feel in control over it all. No brown liquor. No wine until five o'clock. No more than three glasses. These rules were bent and mangled and eventually dropped in the dust, along with numerous empties and a lot of my pride.

I couldn't quit. But I also knew that I would have to, eventually. This was not a situation that could be managed or handled anymore. "Dana sure likes her wine!" had turned into "Dana will die if she keeps this up." I had my brother as proof. I was trapped.

When faced with this horrific reality, I did this: I ignored it and kept drinking. Life or death decision-making just didn't seem important. I would deal with life or death later. There was something much more vital that took precedence: I just did not want to be *bored*.

Using "boredom" as my main argument against sobriety is sort of like someone with a cancer diagnosis refusing treatment because "wigs are itchy."

But oh, how I feared boredom. Life without drinking would be so dull. I needed some sort of daily celebration in my life; the kind that didn't look like a party at all anymore. The kind of party that involved me, a couch, and despair. That kind of party.

When I finally started to tinker with the idea of quitting, I stepped a toe in by saying to myself, "I'll quit for three months. Or maybe two. Just a reset. And then, I'll be all fixed, and I'll just start drinking again, but with a responsible and healthy mindset, like someone who really just enjoys a glass of fine wine.

I'll become a sommelier. You know, I've never really trusted those people who drink for a living and aren't slurring around all the time. But maybe, after this little tiny reset, I'll become that kind of person. I'll talk about alcohol having hints of grassiness or blackberry, instead of just, you know, its ability to annihilate feelings. I could be that person. In two weeks."

You know the story. Two weeks were washed over by the grace of my recovery group and their stories, and after a while, the miracle came and sat in my heart, and I didn't think about time anymore. I wanted to stay here, in Soberland. Forever. And also, one day at a time. I wanted both.

This is sober foreverness. I take it in 24-hour increments. My sobriety needs to be as predictable as the sunrise. Permanence and grace must hold hands. And at times, the concept of forever can elicit a sigh. A stone in a field is permanent, but it's weathered, chipped, and ground down by the elements, and yes, I'm comparing myself to a rock. I'm weathered, y'all. I do get a bit tired of the journey, all this *waves hands in circles* constantly working on myself biz. There's always so much to do for the upkeep of the soul. It's hard. Maybe, though, if it wasn't, it wouldn't be worth it.

I think permanent sobriety is just being interested in yourself long enough to hang around.

Statistically, alcoholics have it tough. I had a 70 percent chance of relapsing, which I did in my third year of recovery. And as "forever" goes, I only have about a 36 percent chance of staying sober forever. Permanently.

Like, that's a really long time.

In my first months of sobriety, I would sit out on the back patio, a big, cold glass of lemonade by my side (I always had some sort of drink with me. It was my wubbie. I discovered the joys of fizzy water and would open a can of La Croix and accessorize it within an inch of its life with cranberry juice, or cucumber slices, or a bag of cheesy puffs. Cheesy puffs pair very nicely with La Croix Lime.) I grabbed every quit-lit book I could get my hands on, and I read and prayed and kept going, one day, one hour, one minute at a time. There isn't a manual about staying sober permanently, what *forever* would look like in Soberland. I wanted one. I wanted a list to print out and affix to my wall, so I could tick items off and feel secure in my foreverness. If there is such a guide, though, I imagine it would look like this:

How to Stay Sober for a Very Long Time: A Manual

Chapter 1: I don't know. Forever is, like, a long time. Let's just stay in the present, OK?
Chapter 2: Calm down about Chapter 1.

The End

Oh, it's a scary thing, permanence. It's the bigness of it. But I loved bigness. Big Feelings. Big Fun. A Big Life, full of Big Meaning and lots of capital letters. So, Big Permanent decisions should fit right in, right? It's dramatic. It's powerful.

It is. But . . . also . . . it could look a wee bit . . . uh. . . Boring?

Let me just clarify: Quitting drinking was the least boring decision I have ever made. It was rebellion. It was a revolutionary act. It was me, waving my La Croix, singing "Do You Hear the People Sing" from the top of a smoky rampart in a French accent! Vive la sober!

And also on some days, it could be boring.

C'est la vie.

About three years ago, I started looking for pretend real estate because TikTok is fascinated with tiny houses and delusional thinking. The videos were impossibly cute and aesthetic and so very *tidy*. I would breathe and watch as a tiny twenty-year-old in her tiny house would open up her sink and do a morning face regimen involving fourteen bottles stored in a cute basket. And then there would be a tiny breakfast involving avocado and sprouted bread, which would be eaten while staring at the forest. Holy moly, I wanted to be there. And not only did I want to be *there*, I wanted to be *her*. I would be in bed watching this[1], as I heard my boys arguing outside the door about who didn't flush, which was always a fun argument to listen to because of the details.

The algorithm kept working its magic. I got sucked into day-in-the-life videos about high-rise apartment owners in New York, where at night you could look out over the city with all its lights and high-up activity and astronomical rent that matched the altitude. Then, there were remote villages in Sweden with snow and big expensive sweaters and hygge-ing[2] all over the place.

I don't know why I started in on these faraway places. Living in an apartment overlooking a big city was never really my thing. "But that would be so *cool*," my brain said, as it viewed a cool white living room with minimal furniture and tall buildings all around. I think what my brain was really saying was, "This is so different from anything I have ever contemplated before in life." My brain liked the difference. I imagine, at 50 years old, it was saying, "I've done all the stuff." And that's when I asked the fun two-part question I had been dealing with since Chapter 2.

Is it depression? Or is it a midlife crisis?

This kind of toggling started with Covid-19, where I would teeter back and forth between: Is it Covid-19? Or just a bad cold?

Was I just bored? Or did I need to find a flat in Barcelona?

I tried this idea out on my friends. "Do you ever just want to, you know, like *go away*?" I blurted while talking with my friend Diane. There hadn't been much lead-in. I think we had been talking about books. "Like, just forget you have a family and somehow they'll all be ok, and move to a small villa in Prague and start working there at a tiny bistro on the corner because they just lost their chef and are desperate. And suddenly you can make good kolache and assimilate with Czech culture, and you have an orange cat that came with the apartment named Jacub (but you change its name to Gary). Also, the apartment has a balcony with a tiny table and chair?" I come up for air. "Oh! And a library! You have a whole wall of books that came with the flat, but they're in English, and it's just you and your cat and all those books and the kolaches?"

Diane sort of stared into the distance. And then she said, "Oh my heavens, *yes*."

The midlife crisis has long been attributed to men and their red cars. Embarking on research about midlife crises culminates in article after article about males. Women just don't seem to have the time, I guess. I once asked my husband if he had ever felt like getting the red sports car or pursuing an affair. "You know . . . the whole midlife crisis thing. Do you ever get bored? Like, with me?"

Brian, ever pragmatic, nodded toward the kitchen wall calendar that is squished full of every sporting event possible because our sons like competition and overpriced gear. He wearily said the obvious: "How would I find the time?" It was a boring answer because you want to be bundled up in the arms of your love when you ask this, and told with a smothering of kisses, how could I even dare to speak of such a thing? But honestly, an affair for me would mean I would have to do a better job shaving my legs. I also don't have time.

The midlife zone is perceived as dull and perhaps even stagnant. It's the least researched of all the age groups, seemingly because we just don't have anything all that exciting going on. I could gently suggest that menopause is suuuuuper exciting, but that's just my plea for help amid all this hormonal sturm und drang. In actuality, middle age is fraught with transformation, especially for women. The Seattle Midlife Women's Health Study spanned over twenty-three years and found that the most challenging part of midlife for women WAS constant change. Changing relationships with partners, children, and aging parents, career fulfillment, and balance are all key stressors for women in midlife. Additionally, women reported that it's the interconnectedness of these stressors that was so tough. We have family responsibilities that are connected to job loss or change that are connected to mental health and finances . . . our lives are so spread over all these relational components that when one thread is plucked, the whole web vibrates. This sort of midlife challenge is perpetuated by the multitasking mom vibe. We can have it all, right?

But also, we're exhausted.

I think it's assumed we should just know the way. And underneath, all the things are rippling with transition. But on the outside, maybe it looks a little boring?

Looks can be deceiving.

Boredom does have a bad reputation. In a really depressing study in 2014, people who were left in a room for up to fifteen minutes chose to administer a self-inflicted electric shock to lessen their time.[3] I would like to point out, however, that only 25 percent of the women in the study zapped themselves rather than just sit there and think their thoughts in the quiet. Men? They zapped in at 67 percent. A lot is going on with this tidbit from science, but I'll stay quiet, else I get snarky. I'll just sit here. With my thoughts.[4]

Neurologically, boredom is just a lack of stimulation followed by a feeling of dissatisfaction. It's almost universally perceived as a negative state, but the general vibe of boredom is that it's awful, but doable, like dental work or small talk.

Now, I am wondering if any child sliding upside down off a couch, moaning "Mom, there's nothing to do. I'm booooorrrreed" has ever responded well to being chirpily reminded: "Only boring people are bored." I have said this to my sons since their inception. I've never observed them rise to the challenge and think, "Well, that's right! I'll just go start a new hobby! Maybe geocaching! Or perhaps I'll visit the library and check out a really large book, and I'll find delight in the written word again!" That's just never happened.

I think that's why I feared sobriety so much. Boredom was kind of all up to *me*.

Listen, it's not so bad being bored. Boredom is a way for the brain to rest and reset. Creativity and problem-solving are engendered by such downtime. And, it taught me trust. I could actually feel bored and stuck with myself, and I would survive.

When my son Henry was a wee lad, we used to play a game called Try to Get Henry to Hide. This was because Henry would cover his face because he was a toddler and could get away with stuff like that without people making fun of him. In Henry's mind, the act of hiding his face was enough. Henry didn't have something called object permanence yet, which is a developmental stage for infants and toddlers. Instead, he just figured he would cease to exist if he couldn't see the things around him. Terrifying, if you think about it, but also cute. As time passed, he finally accepted his place in reality, and now, as a teenager, I remind him about this cuteness, and he rolls his eyes. The teen version of object permanence is also pronounced: both my sons forget that anyone else in the house exists unless it's feeding time. It's not nearly as adorable, and sometimes it involves yelling about how they don't see that they've left dirty socks all over the place (see Chapter 16).

Object permanence directly influences a developmental stage called object constancy. A baby will not emotionally be able to accept that people are the same people over time; the infant only connects the person to whatever feelings she causes in the moment. So, for Henry as an infant, I was Happiness because boobs. I was also Rage because diaper cream, something he was so adverse to that he would bleat at me during each diaper change in tiny infuriation. But as he grew older, he learned to trust that Mom is the same no matter what feelings she causes. Mom is Mom, even when not in the room. And thank goodness, too, because if my sons both equated me to the feelings I create in them now, they would label me Super Cringe. This is totally inaccurate. I am Delicately Cringe.[5]

Adults have learned object constancy. We participate in this weird ratio of knowing "Well, Brian is mad about how I left the door to the freezer open, but also he trusts that I am still the same person I was before I left the freezer door open, which makes it all ok." Something like that.[6]

Let's try to test this theory out on him.

Interview with Brian about the Steak Incident:

Me: Brian. Remember when I left the freezer door ajar?"

Brian: Yes. Can I turn on the game?

Me: Am I still the same person to you, even though I left the freezer door ajar?

Brian: What?

Me: Am I?

Brian: Are you what?

Me: The same! Am I the same person?

Brian: Is this for the book? I feel like this is going to be for the book.

Me: No.

Brian: . . .

Me: Yes.

Brian: Look, I don't want to talk about the Steak Incident anymore. I'm not going to divorce you because of meat. We've gone over this. Hey, that sounds good, though. Want steaks for dinner? Oh wait.

So, all this constancy and permanence and stability, ideas so often paired with words like "predictable" and "same" and "boring"- they're good. They're necessary. But I wonder, am I able to realize this for myself? Am I constant and unwavering to . . . *me*? If I leave the room and leave myself by screwing up, betraying myself by binging out on food for example, am I still me? Am I still to be loved?

Well, of course. But it's good to be reminded. It's like how I tell my boys as they exit the car at 7:55 a.m. for school, "I love you!" Sometimes I even add a "Make good choices!" to see if I can get an eye roll because that's fun. My morning "I love you" is kind of just background music at this point. One kid is already nodding to a friend as he walks past. Another is forgetting his lunch in the car. They hear it, but they don't hear it. But it's still there. It's always there. Sometimes they mumble a "love you too" and shoulder a backpack that weighs more than an air fryer, and they square up with the day and shuffle inside, in their pajama bottoms and alpaca hair.[7]

I need to tell myself, "I love you!" I say, as I shoulder all the responsibilities and predictability and itchy "fleas of life," as the novelist William Styron called it. "Make good choices!" If I walk out of the room for a little while, am I still me when I come back? Yes. Because being fifty has revealed something delightful: I like who I am. I've been with me for a long time. We're friends.

In 2015, six NASA scientists locked themselves into a dome on the side of a volcano in Hawaii and then stayed in that dome for an entire year. It was part of an experiment, the Hawaii Space Exploration Analog and Simulation (HI-SEAS), to test out what it would be like to live on Mars. NASA's goal is for Mars travel to happen in 2030; this was the third type of prolonged immersion test for its scientists. And the number one thing the crew said was a challenge during this year-long adventure? Boredom.

"Bring books," one of the scientists suggested to future volunteers for the program. "Lots of books." I have to admit, I kind of found this comforting. If even supercool NASA scientists can admit to boredom amid this grand experiment, I can too. Boredom is just admitting I'm a little scared that I can't find meaning in the undergrowth. I have to be willing to stick with it and stay curious in this lovely and sometimes monotonous experiment that is me.

And furthermore:

Sometime this year I found what I think is probably the best thing the internet has to offer: The Dull Men's Club.[8]

It's a club for both men and women who take joy in the banal. One of their mottos is "We enjoy safe excitement." Most posts close by stating their shoe size. They like pens a lot, and one of their offshoots is an "Apostrophe Protection Society." There's lots of picture's with that one.

Here are some sample posts:

Wheat harvest on TV. Watched by a dull tot and grandfather. Even the dogs fell asleep.

Weetabix: warm milk or cold? Discuss.

A tire with zero miles on it has a much thicker tread than a tire with 50,000 miles on it. Where does all the rubber worn from the tires go? Why aren't there piles of rubber dust beside every road? Worries like these are a dull man's burden.

Dull people know it is a truth universally acknowledged that a herbal fruit tea doesn't taste as good as it smells.

I play deal or no deal (short game) on Alexa. One free play a day. I'm currently in the mid-two hundreds on the leaderboard with some £500,000. The leader is on some £46 million. I thought I was dull but surely this person takes the biscuit?

Comment: This may be too exciting

Friends, these are my people.

Notes

1. I would like to say to you that I don't think social media and bedtime are a good mix. But I would also like to say to you that I still do it. We're being honest here, and sometimes a good scroll of TikToks about cats and tiny houses is what happens at night. Progress not perfection?

2. Hygge: to live really cozy, with things like candles, blankets, fireplaces, and soup. Because it's Sweden and there's only sun for half the year, it's either hygge or therapy. Or both. But still, it's Swedish, so the blankets are really cute.

3. I really have to wonder about the scientists gathering the data in this study. How did they stay all cool and anti-judgey about some guy who actually chose to push a button and hurt himself over just, oh I don't know, mulling about the weather for ten minutes? Do the scientists prepare themselves for disappointment in humanity when this happens? Do they talk about the people in the lunchroom later? "He lasted like three minutes. What? Like formulating a grocery list wasn't an option? Guys. We are doomed."

4. I once made the mistake of dreamily asking an old boyfriend, "What are you thinking?" after a particularly romantic and intense cuddling session. This type

of question never ends well. It's in the same category as "Do you know what your problem is?" but it's dressed up as affectionate. When I asked this question (and I have never done so since), he responded thusly: "I was thinking that if I ran an extension cable from my stereo to the wall over there and moved it, I could get a much better sound."

5 Charlie interrupts to say "I would just call you 'Old.'"

6 Actually, if he leaves the room he does kind of cease to exist for me because I have a really good book and a cat here, so maybe I have more development to do.

7 What is up with the alpaca hair? Honestly. I know we're supposed to choose our battles, but Henry had carrots the other day for a snack, and watching him chomp made me want to go buy a bag of feed for a dollar and approach.

8 Not sponsored. But very willing.

Bibliography

1 **Statistically, alcoholics have it tough:**
Carmona, Melissa (2024, January 22). Alcohol Relapse Rates: Abstinence Statistics, How to Avoid & Deal with a Relapse. *The Recovery Village Drug and Alcohol Rehab*. https://www.therecoveryvillage.com/alcohol-abuse/alcohol-relapse-statistics/#:~:text=Alcohol%20relapse%20occurs%20in%20almost.

2 **It's the least researched of all the age groups:**
Lachman, Margie E. (2015). Mind the Gap in the Middle: A Call to Study Midlife. *Research in Human Development* 12 (3–4): 327–34. https://doi.org/10.1080/15427609.2015.1068048.

3 **The Seattle Midlife Women's Health Study:**
Thomas, Annette Joan, Ellen Sullivan Mitchell, and Nancy Fugate Woods (2018). The Challenges of Midlife Women: Themes from the Seattle Midlife Women's Health Study. *Women's Midlife Health* 4 (1). https://doi.org/10.1186/s40695-018-0039-9.

4 **In a really depressing study in 2014:**
Whitehead, Nadia (2014, July 3). People Would Rather Be Electrically Shocked than Left Alone with Their Thoughts. https://www.science.org/content/article/people-would-rather-be-electrically-shocked-left-alone-their-thoughts.

5 **. . . boredom is just a lack of stimulation followed by a feeling of dissatisfaction:**
Kubota, Taylor (2016, September 20). The Science of Boredom. *Livescience.com*. https://www.livescience.com/56162-science-of-boredom.html.

6 **Boredom is a way for the brain to rest and reset:**
Robinson, Bryan (2020, September 2). Why Neuroscientists Say, "Boredom Is Good for Your Brain's Health." *Forbes*. https://www.forbes.com/sites/bryanrobinson/2020/09/02/why-neuroscientists-say-boredom-is-good-for-your-brains-health/?sh=76dfebac1842.

7 **Henry didn't have something called object permanence yet:**
Betterhelp. (2024, April 23). "What Is Object Constancy and How Does It Affect People? https://www.betterhelp.com/advice/general/what-is-object-constancy-and-how-does-it-affect-people/.

8 **In 2015, six NASA scientists locked themselves into a dome on the side of a volcano in Hawaii:**
Phys.org. (2016, August 29). Boredom Was Hardest Part of Yearlong Dome Isolation: NASA Crew. https://phys.org/news/2016-08-boredom-hardest-yearlong-dome-isolation.html.

15

Change

When I was in college, Pearl Jam came to our campus and played on the Hill—a large swatch of land with no shade and a whole lot of marijuana. Not growing, but lit. Because I was nineteen and everyone I knew was going to hear this new band, I decided to try something new and tag along. I have to admit I'd never been to a rock concert[1] before. And that's when I found out that I kind of hate them.

No, not "concerts" like when my sons started playing in the orchestra. We attend all of those concerts. Brian and I would turn into those hapless parents in *The Music Man* who, upon hearing their son Timmy blow something out of a horn that made it sound like it was dying, dissolve into rapture. "That's my SON!" we would smile with joy as our kids mangled an orchestral version of Teenage Wasteland because our orchestra director is cool.[2]

No, I'm talking about concerts where you have to stand the whole time, and the band never starts when it says it will. And because you are 5′2″, you only get a good view of the speakers on either side. Also, the speakers on either side? They are so loud.

Now, there are usually about a good twenty minutes in there, when I enjoy myself and sing along, and get all bouncy up and down. But Pearl Jam was a "festival," which meant there were all these acts prior with names like Rage Biscuit and The Nips, and I can't sing along with them because I never smoked enough pot to like their music. Also, it's HOT and I didn't bring sunscreen because no one does. It's the nineties, and everyone is drunk. Sunscreen was not on the list. I am not drunk because beer and heat are not my favorite cocktails, and I'm not an alcoholic yet.³

But I'm trying to have a good time. This is something new, and I'm trying to give it a go. I'm watching some guy dance simply by standing and swiveling his head back and forth, like he's saying "No. No. NO," over and over. Then he vomits onto some girls' picnic blanket, but they don't notice. I want to go over there and tell them, "Hey, this guy puked all over," but it's too late. They thrashed through it, and they didn't seem to notice, so I let it go. Everyone was so sweaty. There's a lot of patchouli. I'm kind of thirsty, but we drank all the beers, and there isn't any water because it's the nineties. Nobody carried around a constant water companion back then.

But oh, how I wish we had.

I got sun poisoning. About four hours into this festival, I started to feel chills and a fever, and then I started throwing up everywhere. I felt like I had the worst flu of my life, and I hated Pearl Jam. To this day, I cannot stand Eddie Vedder's mumble. This is a bummer because Eddie is a great musician. And yet, he nearly killed me.

Since then, I haven't really gone to many concerts. I did go to U2's Zoo tour. It was at night, and if I wanted to sit down, I could.⁴ It was dark, and my friends were nicer.

I also went to see Norah Jones in the early 2000s, but Norah was ok if I sat down. Her music was silky and gorgeous, and it made me feel like it was easier to breathe, like the music was oxygen. Her music made me notice things; the stars when I left the venue were so crisp and bright that we stood looking up for ages, just experiencing them.⁵ So, it was straight-up inspiration smushed into a stadium for two hours. I bought all of her albums after this event, and I am still a huge fan.

In 2013, Norah did a weird thing: she decided to pair up on an album with Billie Joe Armstrong, the guy from Green Day.

Let's go back to that Pearl Jam concert on the hill at KU. If Green Day had been old enough, they would have performed at this festival. Billie Joe had green hair and wore eyeliner and sang into the mic in a way that made you feel angry right along with him. Of course, he did come out with that "I hope you have the time of your life" song, which is earnestly performed at every high school graduation so the parents can cry, but for the most part, Billie Joe is a punk-ass kid. And then Norah Jones, with her long dresses and sweetness, said, "Come away with me," and off they went to make an album together.

Foreverly covered songs by The Everly Brothers, and it was a gentle, sweet rockabilly ode to them. It was also a big detour from both Jones' and Armstrong's style. Since it was a departure, some fans said, "Don't do that. Don't change. This isn't as good as the stuff you always do." *Foreverly* wasn't a huge hit, but for those of us who listened, it was lovely. Different, but good.

Change can be good. But, any sort of change kind of freaks out the brain. It pulls the rug out from under all the set and predictable little patterns the brain employs, and any time this occurs, the brain responds with a "Whoa! ERROR!" signal. Fight or flight is employed. This can be if you see a deer in the road and have to swerve and there's real danger, or if you want to start eating a salad a day because you keep hoovering chimichangas. The brain reacts the same way but with a different ERROR! intensities. It would be super nice if the brain could figure out a more rational approach for all of this, so my amygdala could stop trying to freak me out about a salad, but you know. I guess the brain has enough to do.

I enacted The Salad Rule a few years ago because of Chapters 1–3, and I still follow it today. But for the first couple of weeks, my amygdala kept being very dramatic about it. The prefrontal tried to be rational and interjected with a, "Hey, calm down, it's just salad," but it took quite some time and a lot of energy to adapt to this new salad frontier. It was a change, and change is painful. It was why I didn't want to get up and walk to the library and check out books on birding instead of lying on the couch and watching *Virgin River*. It's why I kept putting off the mammoth project of querying for agents. And, it's why I didn't want to quit drinking, of course. That was fight or flight city for me. Sobriety was way more terrifying than a deer in the headlights, but the outcome looked similar. My prefrontal didn't even try to get all that involved, as it had been stewed in alcohol and was incapable. Perhaps that is why I drank. It gave me permission to not act on my dreams.

But the cool thing about the pain of change is that it can be a *good* hurt. I realize that sounds like I'm a CrossFit junkie who intones, "Pain is temporary. Muscles are forever."[6] But it's true. The tearing down of those highly regulated synapses forces adaptation. Adaptation forces fortification. Change in the brain can create resilience and a sense of well-being. It can help cognitive function and memory. There's no end to all the wonderfulness that is change.

Unless it's awful. Unless, for example, my cat Steve gets sick. And then he dies.

The first time I noticed something was up with Steve was when I took a picture of him. This was not an abnormal occurrence. Steve was my muse, and sometimes there were more pictures of his large white face on my phone than of my children. Steve was a kitten when I started writing for "real," meaning he cuddled me through a fledgling freelance career and then two books. Whenever I would sit down with my laptop, he would thunk up on the table and sit behind the screen, peering over its lid with quiet disdain. "How," he would say with a soft swish of a perfectly orange and white striped tail, "How can you ignore all *this*?" and he would pose. Steve was, shall we say, big-boned. He was a giant of a cat and had the disposition of a bean bag that wanted to cuddle. Sometimes he would walk directly across the keys as I typed and thwak me in the head with his gigantic furry forehead. Then, he would tuck his paws and meatloaf up beside me, waiting for the occasional scritch between the ears.

He never left my side.

I loved that cat. When anyone was upset in the house (which was often because the boys were a lot younger and being upset is a toddler preset), he would get up, look at me as if to say, "Hey, I'll be right back" and he would jump down from the table with a thump and find the child of concern. He would plop down beside them, with a large white belly all soft and ready for a head to lie on. We have pictures of the boys carrying Steve around upside down while he stares at the camera, implacable.

But when I took this picture and then peered at it, I noticed something; Steve looked . . . thin. His haunches were sharper, where once there was only squeezy softness; now he had angles. He was still eating and drinking, but he slept all the time. It's hard to tell with a cat because he slept all the time anyway. But still, I made the vet appointment.

And in about two weeks, he was dead. Steve was first diagnosed with diabetes. I called Brian and sobbed. "He has to be given shots every four hours." I'm pretty sure Brian, somewhere in there, watched this thought roll by: *Why would we give shots to a cat every four hours? This is the time when people like our dads say things like "put down" and "bury in the backyard."* Brian, thankfully, did not allow these thoughts to fully surface, and we embarked on fixing Steve's insulin levels. This involved three more trips to the vet to assess his blood sugar, and the look he would give me while I poked him was so magnificently patient. I would kiss his large head and say, "I'm sorry. I'm sorry," and he just twitched at the pain of it. We kept trying. But he was miserable. He looked miserable. And then he stopped eating, which in Steve's language is pretty bad. We took him back to the vet. They all knew him there. "Hi, sweet Steve," said the vet tech as she took yet another blood sample. "My poor boy."

Molly came in. "It's his liver, Dana. It's just giving out. I don't think . . . " And I looked down at the shrinking warmth of him. Steve looked at me and blinked slowly. He said, "I'm tired."

So, our dads were right. Molly asked if I wanted to wait, but I said no. I couldn't do this to him anymore. When it was over, I cradled his body wrapped in a towel while Brian drove us home, and when I got inside the front door, I howled with pain. And when Brian dug a hole for him by our rose bushes, I bent over and placed Steve on the ground, and then placed my hands on the earth and howled some more. I was keening. I just couldn't stop. My beloved boy was gone, and we had to put him in the ground.

Grief changes. From day-to-day, I would find myself angry, sad, fond, angry again, and dull. I would be numb with exhaustion from missing him, and then I would be exhausted, period, like my whole body ached with tired sadness. I would laugh at something and think "Hey, I'm better!" and then I'd feel the sharpness of loss.

I know. It's just a cat. But pets are so giving, and they specialize in this thing called I Will Love You and Not Ever Do Anything Other Than That. They are painless that way. Until they die, and then you get loaded up on backlogged pain.

Also, there was a problem with the writing. Steve had been my writing companion for ten years. Now, it was just me and my thoughts and no large white softness nearby for a momentary break and a cuddle. Oh, it was so lonely without him.

Grief is change.

And change is grieving.

I got a kitten. My friend Susanna had a litter of them, and we got a gray one that was feisty and cute. Lucy likes surprise attacks. She is ex-army and has a little green beret and a lot of military secrets. She does not like to be touched. She does a lot of skittering. Occasionally, when all the stars align and she is hungry, she will blink slowly and allow someone to pet her, but it's rare. She's so soft and adorable, but it feels like you hallucinated it all, like that whiff of softness was some sort of fever dream. We should have named her Smoke because that's how cuddly she is.

She is not Steve. I kind of wanted her to fill the Steve-shaped hole I've got, but it's so big (Literally. His nickname was Biggie Meows). None of this was fair to Lucy, our sweet psycho-kitty.

One day, I decided to "drive by the animal shelter." By "drive by" I mean I brought home *another* cat. As I did with Lucy, I didn't tell Brian. There was a lot of hustling of food dishes and carriers, and I managed to get Milk all cozy in my upstairs office before Brian got home because Brian is a dog person, as demonstrated by his own annoying golden retriever personality. I figured Brian wouldn't notice another cat walking around upstairs, and I was right. It was two days before he finally came downstairs with a quizzical expression and said, "There's a cat upstairs. Not the gray one. This one is orange." Brian accepted this, and we all adapted to Milk. And Milk is large and orange, and he likes to meow at me at four in the morning. He also likes to grab my hand between his paws, like he's just so excited to see me. It's not Steve-level stuff, but it's cute. Milk and Lucy practice jiu-jitsu in the hallway in the morning, and we adapt to all the fur.

Around the same time that Steve died, I got a tattoo. This was also on a whim, one day after I heard a sermon about Gideon and was inspired by what seemed to be Gideon's rather pronounced insecurities. God would tell Gideon to do big, important stuff, and Gideon kept setting up super elaborate tests and saying things like, "Now, and I'm just checking here, are you POSITIVE you want me to do this?" As I am also insecure, I found this heartening, and so I decided to get a tattoo about it on my arm.

I'm sure I was one of the first people ever to tattoo a bible verse on their body, and I felt very brave. At one point, it was starting to hurt, so I considered stopping the tattoo, but my guy, Mike, had only engraved "Have I not" on my arm at this point, instead of the full verse from Judges: "Have I not sent you?" I tried to think of ways that "Have I not" could work as a life mantra worth carving into my arm, but I couldn't come up with anything.

God is speaking to Gideon in the verse, probably in exasperation. But the tattoo confuses the folks who see it on my arm. They think I am the one saying it, which, to be honest, sounds like something I would gripe in exasperation to my children. But it's God telling Gideon to pull it together and just trust him. "I mean, Gideon, really? All this fleece of the lamb stuff? To dew or not to dew. Can't you just trust me? Have *I* not sent you?"

I happen to identify with Gideon very much.

So one day I drove past a tattoo parlor and I pulled over on a whim and said, "I think I'll get a tattoo today," and that's how *have I not sent you* is now on my arm. Now I can't forget it. I don't ever want to forget that I am not in control. But also? Um, in retrospect? I realize the tattoo is a bit obscure. People think I am the one who is exasperated. I mean, if you don't have any context, the phrase "have I not sent you" is confusing. This, friends, is my life. This is what happens when you do something on a whim and it backfires a little. It's ok. It's not like it's forever, right?

So, also, one day while I was writing at our local coffee shop, a woman came up who works at the library and asked me to apply there. I looked up at Kathy and I thought, "Heck no. I don't have time. I write all day." But, you see, I didn't write all day. I mainly wrote in the morning, and then I puttered about and cleaned something, and there was TikTok scrolling too. "But I don't have time for this," I thought. "I need to write." What I was writing was an occasional freelance article, and then I was also tiredly hitting around another idea for a book. Maybe it would be a novel. I didn't know. My writing and I couldn't seem to get any footing. It was an uneasy feeling. So, I told Kathy I would think about it. I told Brian later that night, "I think I might want to be a librarian." I had been teaching at the local college for ages, but I found myself wanting this, wanting a job with books and quiet and no more endless essays to grade.

Besides, the library gig would be in the afternoon. If I wanted to teach still I could.

I applied and they offered me the job, and here I am, a librarian now. I told the boys, "This will be different. I won't be home when you come home from school. You'll be ok with that, right?" They said, of course, and then they would ask me, repeatedly, where the snacks were when I would get home at 6 p.m. "Mommmmmm I'm STARVING," they would say right as I walked through the door. Look, I am an enabler. I have just enough codependency left in me to know that being home when my kids got home from school was the answer to all of our problems. I had been The Mom Who Was Home for ages. Snack-making was my love language. Providing them with endless cinnamon toast meant love and comfort and maybe a little post-school analysis. This was top-tier Mom behavior. But then, I stopped doing it because I took a librarian job on a whim.

And you know what? After a bit, I was ok with that. The kids were grown. They could make their own damn toast. I changed. We'd be ok. Toast is not the measurement of a mom.

I started doing children's programming at the library. I realize this goes against my "Let's just be quiet and read" philosophy of working there, but it was fun. I was in charge of Lego Club and art events. I thrifted colorful clothes and started posting "fit checks at the library" on my Instagram. My outfits had a Miss Frizzle vibe. I had a vest with cats crocheted on it, and a college kid said it was very "grandma-core." Some days, I wore one of my favorite thrift finds: a t-shirt that says "I'm done peopling" with a mountain backdrop. I don't think anyone was offended by this. The children just ignored it, and most of the older folks felt that way already, so it worked.

And then, there was my hair.

Deciding to go gray on a "whim" is not as quick as it sounds because, you know, it's hair. It wasn't as dramatic or sudden. It's like when, years ago, we were at the airport with two little boys and bags and stress, and we realized that we had to get to Gate Z in five minutes. Brian said, "Let's hop on the cart thing. That'll work." And then when we finally found a car thing, our driver took it so achingly slow I wondered if the universe was just messing with us.[7]

The hair decision was in 2018, before Covid-19, so I like to think I started the trend. Going gray wasn't really because of anything, except maybe a deep weariness about it all. I was always thinking about my hair. I thought about it on a windy day—were my roots showing? I thought about it in pictures. It didn't seem to look right in photographs—my colored hair didn't match me anymore. And I thought about it when I spent a good handful of money on it every three weeks. I was tired of it all. So one day, as I was staring at myself in the rearview mirror in my car, the truthful light of day illuminating every wrinkle and all the freckles, I sighed. I spent so much time covering up. Moisturizer, foundation, and that hair color, all painted on to keep up appearances. And just then I thought, "I quit."

To this day, I get comments. "Oh! I LOVE your hair!" the college girls tell me. "Where did you get it done?" I told them I got it for free, and they exclaimed, "I, like, spent $400 on mine to get it that way," which made me feel freaked out about their finances. I had one lady ask me quietly, "Did your husband mind?" which made me feel really bad for her because Brian had no say in this. I just did it. Also, he calls me the silver fox, and I just love him. Going gray engendered so many comments and reactions from total strangers that I ended up doing a TEDx talk about it.

Also, on a whim, I colored my silver hair purple one afternoon. It was meant to come out a dusty lavender, but instead, it was Barney. I went with it. That weekend, we drove the kids to summer camp, and when I dropped them off, I felt a little bit like Billie Joe. I asked Henry how he felt about his tattooed purple-haired mom. He kind of sighed. "Are you going to get, like, a sleeve?" he asked. I blinked. I had forgotten—oh, a sleeve tattoo—all up and down my arm.

"Probably not, honey. Although I might get one right here," I gestured around my neck. "Like, allllll around my neck. Maybe a tribal tattoo. I'll appropriate someone's culture all up in here." I pointed to my head. "Maybe up on my forehead too?" Henry was silent. "No, I'm not going to do this anymore, I promise. Besides, as time passes, my skin will get more flappy and the message will get folded." He smirked.

In college, my philosophy professor taught me about flux theory. "Heraclitus says, 'You cannot step twice in the same river,'" he lectured. We all wrote this down, nodded, and didn't really get it. Now, I get it. There's change all around me. And the river is still the same.

My recovery changes. My recovery stays the same. And, there's a little bit of grieving with it all along the way. I grieve getting older, the gray hair, the movement of time. I change. And the river flows on.

One day, I decided I'm tired of my laundry room. I paint it pink and add black and white tiles to the floor. About six hours later, it's done. It's lovely. It makes my brain happy. I add pink chairs to our kitchen island and decide that one day, I will repaint the living room a soft blush. I find a pink velvet chair on Facebook marketplace and bring it home in triumph. Our puppy gnaws on it but it's still lovely. My brain feels happier. I'm annoyed at Pepper, but still. Happier.

I look up "impulsivity" to see if I have a problem. I ask my husband about the sciencey stuff. He's an engineer, and whenever I ask him about sciencey stuff, I see him fluff up his feathers a bit and strut right into a long explanation about the change of momentum of an object. His lecture gains momentum because I have granted him a change in motion toward over-informing me, but that's love.

"Impulsivity" then leads me to articles about addiction, relapse, and binge disorders. Researchers have located a specific peptide in the brain linked to impulsivity, which might be linked to future therapies to help hone harmful impulsive behaviors . . . but . . . what about purple hair? Or a silly tattoo? Or a laundry room with diner vibes? In the past five years or so, as menopause and addictive behaviors started to wreak their havoc on my life, did I start doing these goofy little impulsive things as a healthy alternative? Is my brain starting to figure out how to use my powers for good and not for evil?

Maybe these changing decisions in my life are not serious enough to register as impulsive. But they keep happening. I didn't use to be like this. I had to think and rethink decisions, and usually stayed stuck. Static and certain, that was always my safe place. I'm starting to live a life with a regular pattern of change in it. And I think those changes all point back to one thing: the real me underneath. I dunno. Maybe I'm just molting.

A few days ago, I decided to book an Airbnb in a nearby city for three days so I could write. I told my husband about it after the booking, hoping our schedules might align, hoping again it was better to ask forgiveness than permission. We made it work. Writing retreats include vats of coffee and a couple of trips to Trader Joe's for mochi. Usually, there is at least one trip to a vintage clothing store to soothe my brain because writing for hours makes it feel mushy. At the end of day one, I find a thrift store and immediately spy a Kelly green sweater. It has a bright yellow stripe around the collar and looks like something Marsha from the Brady Bunch would wear. It's a little itchy. I don't care. The color feels like a traffic light telling me "Go" and I buy it. At the register, I grab a pair of pink, pointy sunglasses too.

But my coffee shop has changed. Before, it had a lovely deep green ceiling, the same green as my sweater. There were plants all around, and the owner had a refrigerator at one end full of food that had been donated for unhoused folks. They would come and go, grabbing milk or cereal, and sitting in the coolness of the place. They often had dogs who would plop down on the vintage hex-tiled floor, grateful for a break from all this summer heat.

Now, the ceiling is white. The walls have been painted a soft creamy orange. It's new ownership. They had announced it on Instagram. Even the plants were tidier.

And right where the fridge used to be is a large mirrored bar with all sorts of pretty bottles. There's small batch tequila. Artisanal gin. A marble counter with tall black stools beckons in front of all those bottles, where a few patrons hang out with much more expensive coffees.

This is just the type of bar I used to love. The bottles are all so pretty, jewel-like, and promising. I spy coupe glasses that look as delicate as dragonfly wings. I look at it all just a little too long.

The only table available is one right by the bar, because, of course, it is. I park my stuff, extracting my laptop, my notebook, my pens, and paper, but slowly. I'm off. Where is my green ceiling? Where are my flyers about self-defense lessons and poetry slams (not at the same time, but that would be cool) taped on the bathroom door? Suddenly, I feel cross. I don't like this change.

Has my recovery changed at all since those early days in 2014? I know it has. I'm fully capable now of looking someone in the eye and saying, "No. I don't drink" when they ask me whether I want white or red. If they question me further, I tell them I'm in recovery. And my feathers fluff a bit. This is the good part. This is sort of what I love. "Go ahead," I kind of preen, "Ask me, 'Not even one glass? What if it's New Year's Eve?'" I kind of love that stuff now. Maybe I've just gotten more bitchy. The Dana who never really understood standing up for herself back then? Well, she's changed. She's here now.

All these little moments in recovery, where bars jut into coffee shops, or menopause makes me anxious, or springtime reminds me of white wine—those moments are all around me, all the time. The biggest shift is that I'm grateful for them because they remind me of when I fought back against addiction and survived. The biggest change of my life was my sobriety. Marriage and children don't even come close. Or, more accurately, marriage and children are only intact *because* of my sobriety. The only way to survive permanence is to exchange resignation for curiosity.

As I look over my notes, I see a young kid, probably twenty, with a backpack and large headphones. He asks the large table next to me if he can sit, but just then the rest of their squad arrives, and he smiles and backs away. The place is packed. My table is a four-top, and without thinking, I wave at him and point to the chair across from me. I'm pretty spread out, but I quickly move stuff over as he nods silently, sits, and takes out a large iPad. We are sitting just close enough for it to feel a tiny bit weird. He has a nose ring, and a baseball cap covers his eyes as he bends and starts to sketch on the device. We don't talk but work together at our table for about three hours. This is pretty out of my comfort zone; this working with total strangers thing, but I realize it feels kind of nice. Occasionally, he will sit back in his chair and just look at what he's drawing. I do the same, but I try to coordinate it at different times so it's not awkward. I realize that the bar had made me feel lonely, and now this guy is sitting here, and we're working. I'm not lonely. I peek at his sketch. The drawing is abstract, in a soft rust color. I can only see lines and shading. I can't really make it out.

But then, as he sits back once more, he taps the screen and the image zooms out. I can see now what he's creating.

It's hands. It's two large hands, clasping each other.

An Ode to Leslie Coffee Company: A Haiku

Oh my green coffee shop
Why did you have to become
All cool and shit?

Notes

1   Do they still call them this?

2   Insert obligatory footnote explaining that both boys' school concerts bring me to tears every time. They are GOOD. Our orchestra and our band are GOOD. They're amazing. Our directors are GOOD. I'm a fan. I would sell merch for them if I could, huge white t-shirts with "HIGH SCHOOL ORCHESTRA—THE ERAS TOUR" sprawled all over it.

3   Or maybe I was. My alcoholism was laying in wait for me for a long time. Maybe in college. Maybe even before. I don't really know. It's one of those mysteries of addiction that I have given myself permission to not have to figure out.

4   I didn't. It was amaaaazing.

5   There was no marijuana involved; I promise.

6   Please imagine that statement with an Arnold Schwarzenegger accent.

7   True story. Our driver was very nice. But I think he knew it: this wasn't going to end well. With a resigned expression, he laid on that little squeaky horn, but it was crowded, and there was a moment when people were actually walking faster around us that I felt something inside me just kind of shift into acceptance. We were never going to leave this airport. We would just be slowwwwly scooting along in our little car, feeling somewhat ridiculous, forever. But our kids thought it was fun.

Bibliography

1   **But, any sort of change kind of freaks out the brain:**
    Head Heart + Brain (2021). The Brain and Change. https://headheartbrain.com/brain-savvy-business/the-brain-and-change/#:~:text=The%20research%20shows%20that%20people.

2   **But the cool thing about the pain of change is that it can be a *good* hurt:**
    Lee, Soomi, Susan T. Charles, and David M. Almeida (2020). Change Is Good for the Brain: Activity Diversity and Cognitive Functioning across Adulthood. Edited by

Angela Gutchess. *The Journals of Gerontology: Series B* 76 (6): 1036–48. https://doi.org/10.1093/geronb/gbaa020.

3 **"Impulsivity" then leads me to articles about addiction, relapse, and binge disorders:**
Newman, Tim (2019, October 31). Impulsive Behavior: What Happens in the Brain? https://www.medicalnewstoday.com/articles/326862.

16

Flow

In January of 2022, a bunch of citizen scientists discovered a new planet. And then, in a grand act of injustice, they named it TOI-2180 b. This is really not the creative vibe I would go for. If I had been in that group of citizen scientists, the naming of the planet might have gone something like this:

Citizen Scientists Whatsapp group:

Me: LET'S CALL IT SPARKY

Various professors and sciencey people: No. How about TOI-2180 b. It has a certain flair.

Me: Stroke of Venus?

The other guys: No

Me: Jupiter Shmoopiter?

Them: NO.

Me: *tiny voice* William? It kinda looks like a William.

One guy: I had a cat named William Catner.

Everyone: *gasp*

And thus, Planet William would be introduced to the world.

I think creativity is just figuring out how to find lovely things.[1] Lovely things are important. They teach us that there is meaning in the mundane, and they fight off the addicted voice that says, "Let's just zhuzh things up a little."

At the beginning of my son Charlie's ninth-grade year, he was almost late for his first choral concert. Charlie was wearing a tux provided by the school. It was about two sizes too big, and he was muttering a lot, looking for his shoes and bow tie, looking for all the things that made him look suddenly older, suddenly not like my little kid anymore. He was giving off David Byrne Big Suit vibes, but when I tried to explain this to him, he just interrupted, "Why are there NO black socks in this WHOLE house? WHAT DID YOU DO WITH THEM?" which dampened my enthusiasm for him and also for parenting. Charlie had been doing his own laundry for ages, but every once in a while, a glitch in the matrix would occur, and there would be NO BLACK SOCKS ANYWHERE, and that? That was always on me.

Words flew. I started in on Argument with the Kids: Episode #458—I Am Not Your Maid. A full-on three-point lecture about responsibility and socks followed him as we headed for the car, and everything seemed awful. Bickering does that. It sucked the life right out of me. As Charlie slumped in the seat, any sign of expression erased from his features, I'm pretty sure it had this effect on him, too.

I pulled up to the school, and Charlie exited the car without a word, shutting the car door just a teensy bit too hard. I took a deep breath and started in on Negative Self Talk: Episode #245—You Have Failed Again, and trudged inside. The auditorium was nearly full, and I snagged two seats up at the front. Brian joined me about twelve seconds before the concert started because he likes to live on the edge. He kissed me hello, the lights dimmed, and then the singing started. And at one point, I watched my son walk down the risers and approach the microphone. I realized that my son had a solo. He was going to sing a solo. In typical Charlie fashion, he had not told me. He didn't want it to be a big deal.

He started singing. Charlie's voice was strong, deep, and unafraid, and he leaned into the words. He sang the words. He *was* the words. My eyes filled with tears.

Later, I would try to tell him how much I loved his face when he sang, but it got weird, and he mumbled, "Thanks," and that was all. I was awed by him. There was so much more about my kid that I didn't know, that I hadn't seen. It changed me.

Charlie is a creative soul, and his singing is a testament to that. The outer expression of something lovely and true, that's creativity. But also? It's not just output. Creativity is inner work. That moment of kismet, when I saw this true spirit *in* Charlie, mended something in me. Together, we took a beat and found the good and the lovely in the moment. He allowed himself to express it, fearlessly, and I allowed the moment to teach me.

I realize this all sounds rather woo-woo, but I take creativity very seriously. It has saved my life. Trying to explain this is a little like trying to explain faith. You can come off as a wee bit nutball. But I think addicts really get creativity. We have to. We get sober and we get wrung out. There is nothing else. Creativity is all you have. It uncovers who you are, but gently.

Recently, I found myself broaching the subject of creativity with total strangers at yet another coffee shop. I had been writing nonstop for three days, so my brain was sore. It felt overstimulated and precious at this point, like all my ideas were either wonderful or dross, and I had lost the power to discern.

I was on the last day of my writing extravaganza, and I was exhausted. I usually don't sleep well on these trips because I drink vats of coffee, so my weariness perhaps made me step, once again, way out of my comfort zone. I was stuck on a paragraph, so I looked up and took a deep breath, and then I smiled at the other two at my table, "Hi. Is it ok if I ask you something?" They smiled back, and I didn't wait. "Yeah, um. Is creativity important to you?"

This, as you know, is not exactly an easy question, and also, we were just chilling and working; why did I have to be awkward? To their credit, both Nayeli and Morgan accepted my weirdness. Perhaps it's because they are young, both in their late twenties or early thirties. They had an earnest thinkiness about them both that I appreciated, and Morgan actually took notes on what Nayeli said to prepare his own answer.

Nayeli thought for a moment and then spoke. "I come from a background of poverty, and watching the impact it had on my parents . . . they were unable to problem-solve with it. Poverty keeps you stuck, and I think creativity is about being able to think a way out of it. Out of being stuck. I think God gave me that, that ability to rest in him, and then that gave me an open space."

I nodded. "A safe place."

"Yes. All that chronic stress, you just want to survive. It's dis-order. Creativity is order. It's a freedom. God-given."

Nayali shares that they work together at a local church downtown. The website says their church is a "multiethnic community," and yep, right there on the Leadership page is Morgan. At our table, he sits with his notes and stares at them before he speaks as if he doesn't want to get this wrong. I tell him he's not going to, but Nayali laughs. "He likes to think a lot about **all** the things," she says. And so, I wait, and he puts down his pen and says, "The way I see it, by nature we are all creative people. I see it in different cultures, different parts of the world, different perspectives. Jesus was an immigrant on the run. He moved toward the people in the margins. And he found a lot of beauty and goodness in those different places."

So, creativity is beauty and goodness. What a lovely definition.

All of a sudden, Morgan laughs and leans back, like he has the answer. "I mean. Have you seen the movie *Soul?*"

I nod. "That movie made me cry. Animated movies are not supposed to make me cry."

He nods back. "Yeah. I watched it again with my kids about a week ago. And . . . " he trails off. "Ok, I wanna get this right. There's this scene at the end, you know? The big moment for the main character. He has his big night, jamming with all those jazz players, and when it's over, he looks kind of sad." I remember this scene. I've felt like this scene.

"The dude, he like finally made it, you know? This big moment that he had dreamt about all that time. But he's downcast. A woman in the club asks him, 'What's wrong?' and he says, 'I thought I'd feel different.' I mean, he's finally arrived, you know?"

"And the lady, she tells him this parable about a fish. This fish keeps looking for the ocean, asking the fish around him, 'I'm looking for the ocean. Have you seen it?' And this one fish finally tells him, 'Dude. You're swimming in it. You're *here.*'" Morgan smiles.

"So, I guess, that's what creativity means to me. It's finding the meaning and beauty, and goodness in the mundane. The right now. Purpose. *We're. Right. Here.*" He taps the table.

In a coffee shop, I found beauty and goodness listening to those kids tell me about their lives. Something in my heart leaned into their hearts, and we had a moment together at a crowded table. I think they did a better job explaining the importance of creativity than I ever could.

Addiction works in opposition to creativity. Addiction tells your soul, "All those things about you that are lovely and trying to grow? They don't really matter. Shut it down." I listened to that nonsense for *years*. I mean, is it any wonder that the book deals never occurred until after I got sober? Once I got sober, I had the space.

My father will read this book, maybe. And this chapter might make him think, *For Pete's sake, Dana. Always with this. I don't have time for mamsy-pamsy creativity. That's for those artist types. I've got to go mow the lawn.*[2] But my dad is one of the most creative people I know. For example, he is currently mowing his lawn with a machine from 1997. He never throws anything away. He rigs things, like lawnmowers, washing machines, and bank accounts. He never accepts defeat. He has a recipe for duck soup that is top secret and delectable. He makes it every November after serving grilled duck for Thanksgiving. It's a tradition.

Dad's been sober since 1971. He was raised in an era of martini lunches with the big guys and then getting so soused his boss couldn't remember where he left the convertible. We watch *Mad Men* and think it's lore? It was Dad. For him, creativity is just a means of production, of fixing things because that's how he sees the world. The world is a place to be fixed. Or, at least, rigged up with a spare fan belt and some wire.

And my dad has helped so many alcoholics. He has guided and mentored them and helped keep them *alive*. That's creativity incarnate.

When I was teaching high school, I would tell my class, "We're going to get into groups and then creatively problem-solve a way to build a tower out of marshmallows and paper clips" or some such weirdness. I bet the introverts in the class would inwardly sigh and think, *If I hear the phrase 'creative problem-solving' one more time, **I'm** going to be the problem.* Teachers love to make their students try to problem-solve. My favorite example of this was when we had them fill out a "Think About It!" worksheet when they got in trouble. One question asked the kids to reflect on their specific brand of misbehavior.

The worksheet asked: How did this decision impact others?

One kid responded: It didn't. Well, maybe the hamster. Mr. Fluff might be mad, but he got some Cheetos out of it.[3]

My dad would argue that he isn't Creative, with a capital "C," but he is one heck of a problem solver. Researchers have categorized Big-C creativity as genius level, one of prominence and status, and probably recorded in history.

Frida Kahlo and Patrick Mahomes are Big Cs, for example. This is who we compare ourselves to when people ask, "Are you a creative person?" Come to find out, these researchers insist creativity exists on a scale, starting at Little-c creativity and heading up from there. In my opinion, Dad has attained what the researchers call Pro-C status, a highly motivated individual who has wielded innovation, expertise, and hard work into one grand experiment of success. I would so love to see Dad sit down with the students from my class with their marshmallows and paperclips. "Listen," he would say, leaning into them, because he's intense that way. "You, in the weird t-shirt. Sit up. Now, all of you, LISTEN." My dad's very intense.

Then he would lean in further and say, "My buddies and I once put a live cow on the roof of our high school.[4] This is child's play. Pass the marshmallows."

Theorists explain creativity as making something new in an appropriate way. The use of the word "appropriate" is key. I could go out behind my house and start making a fort out of my husband's overabundance of KC Royals Plastic Cups That We Must Handwash, but I'm not sure that's creative. It's just passive-aggressive. Creativity gets the brain buzzing, literally, as it causes communication to zap back and forth between two areas of our brain that don't usually talk to each other. In the left hemisphere, we have the default mode network that helps us remember the past and imagine the future. The right hemisphere is better at executive control, which helps us deliver on the plan. It's not that these areas don't like each other, but getting them to connect is kind of like asking a sonata to wash the windows. Highly creative people show higher levels of connectivity with the sonata and the window. And, all this neuroplasticity builds on itself because creativity can be honed. It can be learned. So, maybe I really had something with all those marshmallow towers. It's not just a trait. It's a skill.

There have been plenty of studies that show that creative expression can have a positive impact on recovery. I know this. In my case, the stickiness of my own shame was combated with creativity. I would write about my pain and all my mess-ups. I didn't plan to tackle shame, but that's where the writing took me, especially at the beginning. It was unpleasant. But I kept going. The more I wrote, the more I wanted to. My writing led me through it.

Those journals still exist on the top shelf of my bookshelf in my office. Every once in a while, I take them down and reread them to be reminded of how I am here now, so very far away from all that, and yet still so very close. It's a testament. It's a how-to manual. Some pages are pocked with tears. Some are a bit more practical. "CALM DOWN, IT'S JUST A BABY SHOWER," one page shouts at me. I take a breath and remember:

Baby shower for a friend: check.
Introversion at level 11: check
Lots of wine and beer: check.
Me having an ok time: check.
Leaving second only to the eighty-year-old grandmother: also check.

I still operate like this with social functions, by the way. It's not just a trait. It's a skill.

Anyhow. It's not surprising that these efforts to work through pain find a home with creativity. It's been demonstrated that when groups brainstorm at the workplace, their ideas are more innovative if each group member first shares some sort of embarrassing memory. Something about that vulnerability allows creativity to breathe easy. "Well," Creativity slaps its hands together excitedly after all the cringe has been aired, "Now that we've got THAT out of the way! Let's do this!"

Creativity can even fortify itself by being attacked. When the creator is shamed for her own work, it's called creative mortification, and it feels just as awful as it sounds. I know this nightmare all too well.

Once, long ago, I wrote something and thought it was rather good. I then sent it to a friend in the magazine business. And my "friend" sent me back an email that went something like this:

Dana, this is embarrassing. I mean, really? I expected better from you.

He continued for about three paragraphs to further explain, but I don't remember his point. I don't even remember what I sent him. I guess it must have been awful? But I will always remember his opening line. Those words sent me right back to my childhood, to being scolded, "I'd be ashamed if I were you," when caught misbehaving. His words clanged around in my head like one of those toy monkeys with the cymbals. I would never improve. I would never be a writer. What (clash) had (clash) I (clash) been (clash) thinking (CLASH)?

I never responded. I allowed myself about a day of shock and self-pity, and fear that I had no chance at ever writing anything of worth. And then I got up and wrote anyway. I'd like to add that I did so with strength and teary courage, and there was a heroic soundtrack in the background that made me feel all Pulitzer-like. But no. I waddled with my writing. I received "We regret to inform you" emails all the time, telling me my writing and ideas were not "right for us at the time" but "please try again" and "Hey, whoa, please don't—oh geez, we've got a crier! Here, take a tissue. It's not PERSONAL, lady." Rejection just hurts.

But here's the thing about creativity, mortified or not. It's still pretty light. It's easy to carry. I can take it anywhere. So I pick it up, and I keep going. And sometimes that's what being creative is all about. Continued forward movement (CFM), no matter what. No matter WHAT.

Here are some things in my life that look like CFM:

1. In the summer of Covid, with the kids at home and despair all around, I created a podcast. It's called *The Neighborgood*, and I think it's still out there, in the podcast stratosphere. I was proud of it. The concept was pretty simple. My friend Jess and I would find folks who wanted to share a story about their lives, and they would tell it in a loose interview format. Our tag was "Welcome to the Neighborgood; it's good here," and we wanted to help people see that while the world was burning, we were all so brilliantly different and yet all very much the same. "Story will save us,"[5] we said at the end of each show.

    Starting up a podcast was not simple. Learning all the tech, especially how to edit and finesse a final product, was only possible after watching about fifty YouTube videos and occasionally pounding the table in frustration. I bought a mic. I figured out how to splice things. I hated my voice but I carried on. My first episode had forty seconds of dead air in it. The show slowly improved, and we got a decent following.

2. And then, a year later, I did another creative thing and let it go. Allowing myself to say, "I did that, and I'm glad. But I don't think it's for me anymore," instead of obsessively hanging on out of obligation or pride, that's a gift.

3. I started journaling again. I pulled out my old friend *The Artist's Way*. It felt like an old recipe book in my hands, falling apart, with coffee stains on the pages, and little notes everywhere. Actually, it is very much a recipe book. Good analogy, Dana.

4. I took a course on book coaching and mentorship. When I started out in this career, I longed for someone to walk me through the mire that is writing a book, understanding the publishing world, dealing with rejection, all the endless questions, and vulnerability of it. I want to help other people write their own books.

5. I started a novel. Yep. It's hanging out on my desktop. I work on it when I can't write about myself anymore, but I'm still writing about myself. My main character's name is Alice, and yes, she has a drinking problem (ok it is kind of about me). I just love her to pieces.

6. Very importantly, I made myself in charge of displays at the library because I guess I had a dream to be the one in charge of making tiny outfits for tiny stuffed animals reading even tinier books titled *The Great Catsby*. For summer reading, I fashioned a mountain out of books and strung up a workable zipline, and fashioned helmets out of one-half of an Easter egg. Safety first. This makes sense because we librarians like to live hard.

If I ever quit writing, I have a real future in the art of making costumes for stuffed animals. It's a bit of a niche, but give me a glue gun and some cotton balls and I'm unstoppable. I'm getting *paid* for this. It's a ridiculous joy. There were no extenuating circumstances. The library director didn't come up and say, "Dana, you need to make a Hawaiian shirt for a cat out of fabric scraps and a stapler, right now. This is a library emergency!" Instead, I have a super patient boss who walks past me as I'm trying to figure out how to make crutches out of popsicle sticks for my bunny, Tiny Tim. She pauses for a moment, takes it all in, and then goes back to work. Should I be working on book inventory? Yes. But God bless us, everyone I also made Tiny Tim a widdle tiny hat.

7. Color. My house and my wardrobe look like Willy Wonka and a grandma had a baby. This sounds so icky, but I don't know how else to say it. There are a lot of granny blankets and pinks all over the place. I have dining room chairs with cats on them that I got from an estate sale down the block. I made my sons help drag them back to the house, and Charlie kept protesting. "CAT chairs? Mom, like, are you ok?"

8. I muster some bravery and decide to start running again. Running boosts creativity. The endorphin rush, the flushing of stress—all relate directly to increased creative space in my brain. But what also happened with the running was a sweaty assurance that I could do this hard thing, this crazy return to something that I had decided was impossible after menopause and Covid. I started small, which is not my normal route with anything, but something in my heart said, *Don't be all-or-nothing anymore, Dana. Just . . . be. Just take it a block at a time.*

Deciding to fight back to running again was a courageous thing, and creativity takes real courage too. So, that was me, huffing and puffing and taking it slow. I refused to track miles. I never checked my weight on a scale, either. I still don't. I wasn't doing this for weight loss or to sign up for a 5K. I just wanted to feel strong again. To feel free. Haruki Murakami's playful little book "*What I Talk About When I Talk About Running*" describes the "nostalgic silence" of running, which is right. It's exactly right. The Goodreads reviews of Murakami's book are kind of hilarious, because so many reviewers are complaining that this book never explains the "How tos" of running. Well, yes. The book is a philosophical treatise about the blessed space that running gives him. It doesn't talk about split times or how to deal with shin splints. It's more than that. It's just so much more than that.

When I run, I run right back to myself, the real me, underneath all the noise of the world. That delicious power-down of my brain while on a run? That's the BEST. It was a high that I cannot accomplish pretty much any other way. It was a daily emptying out, a discovery of a clean, creative space.

Maybe that's why I like creativity so much. *It numbs me the heck out.* But, in a good way.

In the spring of 2021, I taught an honors college class about creativity and the brain. My class roster was all girls. I was assigned two books: *The War of Art* by Stephen Pressfield and *Flow: The Psychology of Optimal Experience* by Mihaly Csikszentmihalyi. We spent the rest of the semester just trying to pronounce Mihaly's name. We did some other stuff too.

Pressfield's book is thin. It's about the size of a Jodi Picoult chapter. But each little section, about resistance and fear, thrums so strongly within us all that we take notes, scribble, dog-ear pages and endlessly discuss. Art is necessary. Art is *work*.

Resistance tells us:

You're too old.

It's too late.

You're not worth it.

This stuff is stupid.

Doing something just for the sake of joy? Ridiculous.

Where's the payoff? What's the pay grade?

Or, you're getting paid? Well, that's not art.

Go consume something. Comfort yourself.

This is too hard.

This is too easy.

What are you thinking?

I mean. Honestly? When it comes to creativity? Often, I'm *not* thinking. The zone of flow, according to Csikszentmihalyi[6] is a rather delicious unconscious space. It's an elegant focus that keeps the brain still, but the heart moving. It's medicine.

Flow is achieved when the click happens. Let's say I'm mowing the lawn. But in my head, I'm directing the orchestra for ELO's "I'm Alive." Which one is present and accounted for in my head? The swell of the violins, or the yard? I'm not sure. But the yard mowed itself.

Flow is an uninhibited focus. It's fully *autotelic*. *Auto* = self. And *telos* = end. Or goal. Listening to the self, or the soul, is the only goal.

I try to explain this to my class of highly driven juniors and seniors who have done nothing for the past few years but get the points, the grades, the recommendations, the internships, the vision, while working lousy part-time jobs and submitting endless papers, tests, and an avalanche of assessments.

"True happiness," I tell them, "Is found in doing it for yourself, not for the grade." They take notes. They wonder when the quiz will be. They don't trust it. They certainly don't trust me; I'm the grade giver. "Well, that's what Big C says," I add, realizing too, that this all sounds kind of silly. I mean, does flow buy groceries? Does it pay car insurance? I try again. "You can achieve flow anywhere. In any situation. If you have clear goals and the activity has a bit of challenge, flow can be achieved while you mow the lawn!" They blink.

One of my students, Riley, tentatively asks, "Isn't that just, like, daydreaming?" And, I'm stuck. I mean, she might be right. Perhaps my inner backup singer for Pink is just a sort of glorified mind trip. I do tend to Walter Mitty myself out of washing the dishes, too.

Riley's question worried me about the rest of the semester. Where were we going with this? "And," Callie pipes up, "I keep trying to get there, you know? With 'flow'?" She air quotes, and I feel hurt. "Like, how do you DO it?" They all nod, and one kind of scrunches up her face like she's trying really hard to . . . flow. They want a list of steps. They all gaze at me, expectantly.

So . . . that's where the puppies come in.

In the next class period, I bring a cute wicker basket of puppies to class. My friend Erica is amazing because she did this when I texted her:

Me: Don't you have puppies right now?
Erica: Yep!
Me: Can you bundle them up in an aesthetically pleasing way and bring them to my college class?
Erica: Yep! What's it for?
Me: I have no idea. I just feel like they need puppies.
Erica: Doesn't everyone!?

The class fell silent when Erica walked in with her basket. I think they were in shock. The girls, not the puppies. It's like Paul Rudd[7] just walked through the door. There's a gasp, and hands go to faces, and one girl starts fluttering them at her eyes like one of the puppies just proposed to her.

Erica and I place a puppy in each of the girls' arms. These girls? They didn't get a prom. They didn't have a high school graduation. Covid decided that for them. And that day, I hadn't tied the puppies to the books we were reading, or the curriculum, or, God help us, any sort of outcome or standard. I just wanted them to have some puppies for an hour. Puppies ran around and no one peed in the corner. Time stopped, and puppies took over.

But at our next class, I had questions. I asked them how the rest of the Glorious Day of the Puppies had gone. They visibly relaxed, and I swear all of them smiled, which is kind of a minor miracle when it comes to college kids.

"I felt, like, so chill."

"My next class was actually not boring?"

"I dunno. I called my mom, though."

We all decided together that while we were holding onto those puppies, nothing else existed. It was flow, in a furry way. And just a little bit of that, every day, was all we needed. The girls and I made lists of ways to accomplish flow in our daily lives. "Go for a run," I said. "Music, but singing to it," offered Riley. "Lesson planning," offered another, and I nodded, excited. That creating moment, when I planned lessons for my high school classes—that was flow. "Working outside!" said another. "We live on a farm, and when I go home and help my dad with the chickens and cows? I didn't realize it but it's like my brain just relaxes into it!" What she is describing is something called the "soft fascination" that nature can elicit. It's not mindless and passive. It's that delicious sweet spot where skill level, attention, and challenge hold hands.

We all have access to flow. But it's not a passive activity. It takes a little work and a little practice. Flow also plays well with others. It's experienced best when it's communal. This is such a recovery thing. Recovery is not meant to be done alone. Recovery IS community. It's like the proliferation of roundabouts we see now in traffic. Roundabouts lessen the chance of a crash by up to 90 percent. We slow down; we flow together, yielding in concert with each other. It's safer this way. We are all searching for a smooth roundabout. And it's so rewarding to see it and achieve it together.

Flow amplifies joy.

When I lead a recovery workshop, I like to conclude with some practical ideas for the attendees to have an immediate takeaway. I write a list: "Practice your 'Yeses' and your 'Nos'" and "Stop thinking about getting from here to there," and "Nobody is watching."

And then I share my final point:

EMBRACE WHIMSY.

I SUGGEST PETS AND CHILDREN.

Which leads me to . . .

Notes

1 This includes us. You. Me. We are lovely.
2 But he will think of it in a sweet way.
3 No hamsters were harmed. He wanted to take the hamster into social studies class and he did so, via his pocket. The hamster did not care for that, and the teacher was not emotionally prepared.
4 To this day, Dad has never explained how he managed to do this, but I'm sure there's a physics lesson in there somewhere. #legend #thecowwasok
5 I still believe this. Why do you think I write about recovery so much? It saved me.
6 I really love this guy, but I will never be able to pronounce his name. We all referred to him as Big C for the class.
7 Well, I guess I need to insert a Gen Z heart throb right here. I should know at least one, right? I feel like I should know at least one. But so many of them seem kinda pale and scrawny, and to me they all kind of blend.

Bibliography

1 **In January of 2022, a bunch of citizen scientists discovered a new planet:**
Howell, Elizabeth (2022, January 16). Strange and Hidden Jupiter-Size Exoplanet Spotted by Astronomers and Citizen Scientists. *Space.com*. https://www.space.com/hidden-exoplanet-discovery-tess-citizen-scientists.

2 **Researchers have categorized Big-C creativity as genius level:**
Helfand, Max, James C. Kaufman, and Ronald A. Beghetto (2016). The Four-C Model of Creativity: Culture and Context. *ResearchGate*. Palgrave. https://www.researchgate.net/publication/312854338_The_Four-C_Model_of_Creativity_Culture_and_Context.

3 **Theorists explain creativity as making something new in an appropriate way:**
Tikkanen, Marjo (2019, February 26). Creativity Is Just Putting Things Together. *Medium*. https://medium.muz.li/creativity-is-just-putting-things-together-69f421877c96.

4 **There have been plenty of studies that show that creative expression can have a positive impact on recovery:**
Sack, David (2017). 7 Ways Creativity Supports Addiction Recovery. *Psychology Today*. https://www.psychologytoday.com/us/blog/where-science-meets-the-steps/201710/7-ways-creativity-supports-addiction-recovery.

5 **... their ideas were more innovative if each group member first shared an embarrassing memory:**
Ayshford, Emily (2019, December 2). Why Your next Brainstorm Should Begin with an Embarrassing Story. *Kellogg Insight*. https://insight.kellogg.northwestern.edu/article/boost-creativity-brainstorm-embarrassment.

6 **... it's called creative mortification and it feels just as awful as it sounds:**
Pringle, Zorana Ivcevic (2020, March 12). Managing Emotions to Innovate. Psychology Today. https://www.psychologytoday.com/us/blog/creativity-the-art-and-science/202003/managing-emotions-innovate.

7 **Running boosts creativity:**
PermissionToPlay (2020, September 21). How Running Gets Your Creativity Flowing. https://www.permissiontoplay.co/fieldnotes/how-running-gets-your-creativity-flowing/.

8 **It's fully *autotelic*:**
Akbari, Morteza, Mozhgan Danesh, Azadeh Rezvani, Nazanin Javadi, Seyyed Kazem Banihashem, and Omid Noroozi (2022). The Role of Students' Relational Identity and Autotelic Experience for Their Innovative and Continuous Use of E-Learning. *Education and Information Technologies* 28 (2). https://doi.org/10.1007/s10639-022-11272-5.

9 **What she is describing is something called the "soft fascination," that nature can elicit:**
Gallardo, Luis (2022, January 28). How to Enter the State of "Soft Fascination" and Ultimate Healing. *World Happiness Foundation*. https://worldhappiness.foundation/blog/happiness/how-to-enter-the-state-of-soft-fascination-and-ultimate-healing/.

10 **Flow also plays well with others:**
Oppland, Mike (2016, December 16). 8 Traits of Flow according to Mihaly Csikszentmihalyi." https://positivepsychology.com/mihaly-csikszentmihalyi-father-of-flow/#flow-friends.

11 **Roundabouts lessen the chance of a crash by up to 90%:**
Eustace, Deogratias (2023, October 25). What Are Roundabouts? A Transportation Engineer Explains the Safety Benefits of These Circular Intersections. *The Conversation*. https://theconversation.com/what-are-roundabouts-a-transportation-engineer-explains-the-safety-benefits-of-these-circular-intersections-215412.

17

Are You Any Fun?

I am at a wedding reception. Usher's *It's Getting Hot in Here* starts up, and all the fifty-year-olds start bobbing their heads. My husband is off in search of a drink for me, and I sit quietly, arranging my face into a generic reception-table-smiling, trying not to be introverted. It's awkward, in that wedding kind of way, where a lot of strangers are seated together to celebrate the happy couple. It is still a good time, right? We're all adults here; we can have a good time with strangers.[1]

I breathe in and look around for Brian. He's nowhere in sight. The table members are two couples who know each other, but finally, one woman with a chunky orange statement necklace looks over at me and smiles. "So, how do you know the couple?" she asks, and I tell her the bride is a friend of my husband's. "I'm here as his emotional wedding support wife," I say, and they don't laugh. I start folding my paper napkin into squares and then spot Brian, approaching with the non-alcoholic wedding reception MVP: Diet Coke and lime. Statement necklace says, "Is that their signature cocktail? I was hoping it would be something fruity." I shake my head no.

Brian enters the chat. "It's just a Coke," and the "just" kind of irks me.

"Are they out of wine?" She looks anxiously over toward the bar at the far end of the room.

"I don't drink." I take a sip of my Coke and feel the bubbles fizz at my nose.

There's a beat of silence. "Wow. Good for you," Statement Necklace blurts, like I have announced that I have the moral upper ground. We all wither a bit because whenever anybody announces they have the moral upper ground, it's never good, morally or otherwise. Maintaining eye contact, she slowly clasps her hands around her plastic cup of wine as if to say, "Hey. That's not here." I wonder if she thinks I'm going to lunge for it.

The guy next to her just snort-laughs. "Wait. Really?" Then he leans in a little further and says this: "You know, that's awesome. Good for you, really. But, I mean . . . Do you have any fun?"

This conversation never happened.

Well, that's not true. This conversation did materialize in my imagination, repeatedly, during my last gasp of addicted drinking when I was desperate for any excuse to keep me from giving up alcohol. In reality, this awkward exchange never occurred, but I always imagined it would. My squishy alcoholic brain was searching for anything to land on that could keep me immersed in wine. "Fun" seemed to be a good thing to worry about while I was waking up sick and achy and hiding vodka in my closet. Alcohol was "Fun." Without it, life would be "Not fun." It's math.

Now, I almost wish this couple in my head would find me. I go to weddings and dinner parties and look around for them as I wince-sip my La Croix because LaCroix hurts a bit going down.[2] I sit down, place my glass with a thunk, and smile at everyone. *Come on*, I think. *ASK ME WHAT I'M DRINKING*. Nobody does, of course, because people are nice. Also, one of the first shocking things I learned in recovery is that most folks are not as invested in my beverages as I thought. But anyhow, I still wait. To this day, I am waiting for some guy to ask me after I announce: "I don't drink."

"That's awesome. Good for you, really. But, I mean . . . Do you have any fun?"

Yes.

Every morning when I wake up, I am greeted by Milk, my BOC (Big Orange Cat) who head butts me and does this one long, raspy "MOWWW" to tell me it's time for breakfast. Milk's "MOWWW" sounds like he has a three-pack-a-day habit. He came from the streets, and I'm sure he's seen things. When we first brought him home, he tried to be sweet, but he was always on a swivel, eyes and ears, and whole body tense, ready for danger and always, ALWAYS looking for food.

Now, Milk has a life of luxury, but he remains vigilant. This is because we also have Lucy, the ninja cat, whose love language is attack. I get up, kiss Milk on his forehead, and walk down the hall. Lucy greets Milk with her usual: rearing up on her hind legs, she gives him a right hook to the jaw. Milk responds with a series of soft punches to her ears. This continues, with them standing and swiping, then taking a few steps, weaving and jabbing, until they make it to food dishes where Milk sits and blinks at me. Lucy does a final sweep with her paw and then sits too. They grin.

They are playing. Milk is fully grown; he has no kitten left about his large haunches and big ol' pooch, but he plays now. His fur is glossy and the exact color of a Halloween pumpkin. His eyes are yellow, and they gleam. He is curious, and he's happy.

He plays, and then he sleeps, and then he eats. That's his day. I envy him. It's his reset. When the scary stuff went away, play became his natural state. He loves our little fishing rod toy, and he can't get enough of those poof balls I keep buying so he can bat fifty of them under the couch. He attacks paper bags with so much glee I can almost hear him say, "I GOT you!" He plays even more than Lucy, it seems. She watches him, paws tucked in breadloaf mode as he zings at a bouncy ball with orange abandon.

Play is biological. It's a necessary part of our maturation: through play, we learn trust and persistence. We learn to trust that we are a good time. When we're four years old and we find a really great stick and it becomes a wand, we're doing it naturally. Endorphins release. We practice collaborating with others. Have you ever watched children when they're released outside for recess? They *run*. They don't all stand at the door and ponder all the choices of the playground. They don't comprise a list and then explain: "Well, I think I'll start with the tetherball for a warmup to increase my heart rate, look for bugs under the tree, and conclude my time by chasing Dax. He is available for chasing in *checks watch* seven minutes."

The kids just *go*. It's entirely autotelic and awesome.

"Well that's just *great*, Dana," you say, while you're filing your taxes and taking the dog to the vet to have his anal glands dealt with because he keeps scooting apologetically on the carpet, and then scheduling an argument with your spouse for 9 p.m. tonight. "That's so *fun*. But some of us don't have time for that anymore. You know, because we're ADULTS." It's true. We grow up and play is just smacked right out of us.[3]

And also: Come out, come out wherever you are, Play. We need you.

"Long-term recovery" sounds so *serious*. So does "sobriety." Like, literally. When I sobered up, I had a metric ton of immaturity to work out. It's true that when you finally get sober you're emotionally at the age where you started drinking abusively. This put me, as a mom of two young boys, at around twenty-two. This was horrifying, but sometimes also really fun. And the thing is, I didn't have to banish the immaturity. I just had to channel it.

What we must learn to do in life is use our weirdness for good. So, as my recovery strengthened and lengthened, my inner goofball flourished.

And good for her. I'm proud of my inner goofball. She showed me how to pay more attention, to finally listen to myself, and match my insides to my outsides.[4]

Playfulness came back in bits and pieces. Some days were grim and hard and triggered, and I would go to bed and lie there and cry silently until tears pooled up in my ears. Brian would crawl into bed, notice the cistern on my pillow, and ask the obligatory, "What's wrong?" I wanted to look at him and just say, "I'm an alcoholic!" But I'd try to come up with something more specific because if I didn't, there would be follow-up questions, and I was so tired. He does have the ability to ask just the right question at just the right time to set forth more tears. It's his way.

But recovery is a prism in a window. And there were other moments, lots of moments, where the sun hit just right, that life was so illuminated with joy that I had to stop and stare. It was all a glorious surprise.

About a year into sobriety, I was brave and decided to go out to dinner with Brian at one of my drinking restaurants. People in recovery know what a drinking restaurant is. The Renaissance used to be almost a monthly venture for us because, for Brian, they had excellent pasta, and for me, they had cheap wine. But now, I was going for their artichoke bruschetta.

This restaurant had been off our list of options after I got sober. It just held too many memories of candlelit, highly functioning drunkenness. I had no idea that an entire restaurant could be triggering, but that's recovery for you. Brian would say, "Hey, let's have a date night. Wanna go to Renaissance?" and I would shudder and get mad at him for his insensitivity when he was just aiming for romantic. This made date night fun.

But now, he didn't suggest it; I did.

The restaurant is an old public school building, and we were seated on an upper balcony over the gymnasium. The walls were covered with old photographs, and Dean Martin sang. As our waitress brought in sparkling water (lots of lime) and a small plate of an appetizer, I smiled across at Brian. This was a good decision, coming back. I looked at the little plate before me of what looked like three creamy balls of mozzarella or perhaps goat cheese, rolled in fresh herbs. Renaissance always provided a small bite before dinner on the house, and I was starving. I reached out and popped one in my mouth. And chewed. And then stopped.

It was butter. I had just shoved a golf ball of butter into my mouth. At that moment, the waitress deftly put down a basket of bread. "Here you go. This is right out of the oven to go with your freshly churned butter-" and she looked at the butter plate. She looked at Brian. And then she looked at me. I nodded, frozen, just me and my butter.

She said, "Well. Enjoy?" and then walked away.

Possible kitchen conversation: "Dudes. Butter-eater. Table 7."

I kept chewing, and then, to my horror, I realized the butter was spicy. Like, really spicy.

My eyes filled with tears, but not so much from the heat but from total mirth.

Brian watched me in awe. "Ibs bubber" I said, heroically still chewing. You would think it would have melted by now, but this was a lot of butter. "You shoub try it."

And then I laughed and laughed. It was kind of a greasy cackling, really. It was like I just launched myself into laughing, and did so for about a good three minutes, to the point of tears. Brian, who is a golden retriever, laughed too. He saw me crying in helpless butter asphyxiation and he started laughing along. Twenty years of real laughter had been bottled up inside me, and that day, on that balcony with my butter, I let 'er loose.

Kitchen conversation: "Guys. Table 7. They're on drugs."

But, you see. I'm *not*. And it's hilarious.

Ok, sobriety is not oodles of fun all the time. Not even close. But the laughter and the fun that I now subscribe to is the main line kind. Honestly? I didn't expect to be having this much fun.

It was all a total surprise.

Philosophers have tried to pin down a measurement and definition of what "information" is, and a main theory is that information is simply a unit of the unexpected. All information is surprise. It's what helps us have a deeper understanding of our world. Every time we take in information, the more surprising it is, the deeper we process it. Teachers know this. Any teacher who has pulled up a PowerPoint titled *Please Stop Writing Without Any Punctuation*[5] knows that a bit of surprise might help this situation be more palatable. Surprise can shut down all of the brain's other functions except the area devoted to reward. Dopamine is released, and the brain goes through a kind of astonished reset to focus only on the surprise and understand it better.

Now, understandably, if a tree branch thwacks you in the face as you walk past it, this is also a surprise, and the brain is startled into focusing on that, too. Surprise can be quite unpleasant. The brain doesn't judge. The nucleus accumbens, the reward area of the brain that lights up due to surprise, is also where addictive cravings are generated. Back when I was drinking, my nucleus accumbens was a mess. Honestly, it was just barely getting by. My brain was in an endless wonky loop, set off by repeated addictive behaviors and faux reward messaging, and then its circuits would jam up or backfire, spurting out all sorts of cravings for alcohol. It was a horrible cycle, one that got dizzyingly more powerful with each rotation. It's tough to jump off the merry-go-round[6] when it means you're going to have to fling yourself onto the hard ground. Might as well just shut your eyes and cling harder.

So, it's important to keep the brain functioning properly.

Enter: Fun.

Fun loves a surprise too. Even as a proud member of the Dull Women's Club, I can attest. Getting into bed at 9 p.m. every night to read the new Louise Penny mystery might not seem like the essence of surprise, but it is for me. Attempting a new recipe for banh mi? Asian fusion fun. Going out with my friends at night to dinner every once in a while? Forced extroversion fun. Playing fetch with our linebacker-puppy? Slobbery fun.

Tiny moments of fun, like little bubbles of effervescent reset for the brain: Medicinal, Dynamic, Very Necessary FUN.

Sure, Dana, you think as you attempt a response to Linda in HR's last communication, the one that started with "Per my last email." *Sure, I'll get right on Fun. Maybe I'll invite Linda out to pickleball. It will be So. Much. FUN.*

Well, if you put it that way.

When I was about two years sober, we signed Henry up for T-ball. This was the best decision I have ever made.

Watching a kid named Dax hit the ball off the tee and then run out and *retrieve his own ball* is fun. If any kid hit ANY ball, the entire team would abandon their positions and ALL start running toward the ball. I could almost hear them saying "mine mine mine mine" like a bunch of possessive ducks. Sometimes, kids in the dugout would also get involved.

My kid had a helmet so large it wobbled every time he ran. He was Dark Helmet from *Spaceballs*. He loved that thing. The first time he got a hit, he ran in a straight line right out to second base. It was glorious. One kid started playing on the opposite team, and nobody noticed. He was in the outfield picking dandelions.

I spent a lot of time laughing that summer. Each game was like an improvisational comedy show. We never knew who was going to be the headliner, but all that laughter cleaned me out, like some sort of laughter-colonic. This sounds weird, but also, don't we all just need that right now?

Somehow, getting sober taught me to get a little less serious. My husband is my muse in this category, and he's not even an alcoholic. He's just immature. One of his favorite versions of fun is participating in some insanity called Bike Across Kansas, where he and 400 other weirdos ride horizontally across Kansas *in June*. The BAK has never even considered a vertical "acrossing." I salute them. Each day, these people go on a 20–80 sweaty cycling leg, and afterward, they all sit around and sweat and talk to each other about it. It's horrible. Some opt to sleep inside the school gym, where it's air-conditioned and you can snore along with a couple hundred of your dearest friends, but Brian is too tough for that. He sleeps outside in a tent with the bugs and the heat, and oh my heavens, how in the world is this fun? But, it's Brian-fun. He owns it fully. He plans it every year. He takes off work for it. And this year, as we got up early to drive to his starting point, he looked at me with total glee and said, "Guess what I get to do today, honey?" I mumbled something about sleeping more. He answered: "I get to go on a bike ride!"

And ride, he did. When he got home, with a terrific farmer's tan and a whole lot of really fascinating stories about riding a bike, I realized something: This man takes fun seriously. He had a glow about him, not just brought on by the sunburn. He schedules this fun every summer, and it makes him feel strong. He's known on the ride by many as the "howdy-howdy!"[7] guy, cheerfully greeting fellow bikers as he passed them. Gleefully spandexed, my husband banishes fear.

When Henry was in fourth grade, he was at a friend's house, and the big sister had the marvelous idea to start watching the movie *It* with her friends. The children all did that thing where they could run outside to play in the wholesome sunshine, but oh wait, there's a TV. Transfixed, they gathered. As Henry told me later, "Mom, I tried to come up with an excuse to get out of there, but everyone..." and he kind of shrugged helplessly. Henry hates horror movies, and at that point in his young life, I don't think he had seen anything at this level of scary. He used to get freaked out by Bob the Tomato from *Veggie Tales*. He's a sweet kid. So, this whole "Hey let's watch this terrifying clown movie in the living room" scenario was not ok.

When Pennywise made his first appearance, Henry said to the group, "Well, my mom needs me." And he just stood up and walked right out the door. I have never been so proud.

Pennywise kept coming back, though. Henry had nightmares about this clown for at least a month. When we were talking it over and I was silently deciding this kid would never get to play at a friend's house again, I made up the Boop Rule.

The Boop Rule is simple.[8] I told Henry to imagine the subject of his fears and go up to him or it, and boop its nose.

Boop.

Booping works in all areas of life:

1. I could boop Jaws, and he would kind of wrinkle his cute widdle nose and turn into Disney Jaws, and we would cavort. Or maybe he would just swim off and eat someone else. I don't remember.

2. I could boop the insurance person on the phone, telling me they're not going to cover my hearing aids because I was too young to have them. Boop.
3. W-2s? Still don't remember if it's a 0 or a 1? Boop.
4. My kid starting driver's ed? BIG HUGE BOOP.

That's what fun is, really. It's just a response to fear. It's a gentle answer, like when you're a kid and you're terrified of the drain in the tub because you saw a shark the size of a pickup at a drive-in. Fred Rogers made a song for this very thing, aptly titled *You Can Never Go Down the Drain.* This was a man who understood the power of the Boop Rule. Fred Rogers' gentle accuracy—to name fears, to say them out loud—is why people still talk about this man. He had such a way of easily explaining how we interpret feelings. People have even termed his calm way of shining light on fearfulness: "Freddish."

What would Fred Rogers say about getting older? About waking up in the middle of the night and not being able to breathe? About addiction? I wish he were able to make a song for me titled "You're Not Dead Yet and Your Life Does Have Meaning," or "All the People in the Neighborhood Don't Have to Like You" with that trolley dinging in the background.

Fear is essentially about scarcity. As one who struggles with addiction, I really don't like scarcity. My fears about getting older and sliding off into obscurity are all about the scarcity of time. Time wasn't something I thought about much in my twenties unless it was actual clock time and I was late to work. But as I got older, time seemed to speed up. I would hear my mind tell me: "You're running out of time. You should have started this book sooner, this project sooner, this whole recovery thing SOONER. Why did you waste so much time?" I knew these thoughts weren't productive, and I was right where I was supposed to be, but still. Time seems a lot more slippery now.

This is normal, by the way. As we age, we don't have as many "new" images to process, so time works more quickly. There are, literally, fewer surprises because we've done a lot of stuff. Time slips past us. It squeezes right on by without so much as an "Oh excuse me," and then poof, it's gone. Or at least it feels that way. It's a scary thing to feel that time is running out. Turning fifty might do that. It might tell me, once in a while, "Well, you know. It's all downhill from here," and fear will grumble and commiserate.

What if, instead, I was able to say, "Yes, ok, but let's just stop and take a look here? Let's just get curious for a moment." Life now has a road trip mentality. Like, if there is a billboard announcing that the next town has The American Museum of the House Cat, you take the exit.[9] You *always* take the exit.

Sobriety led me to pursue whimsy with the same energy I had in my twenties when pursuing men. Go ahead. Ask me which energy had the better payoff.

Why fun? Because it's joy training, and it doesn't pay attention to time. My boys have baseball practice, and Brian goes to choir practice. I attempt a meditation practice or the practice of prayer. Why not have a fun practice? Fun is joy with training wheels on, and it's good to keep it toned, like the muscles that are willing to take me on a three-mile run every morning, miraculously. My fun muscles are just as important.

When my boys were little, they were obsessed with the planets and our solar system. They watched a lot of PBS. I had a large glass jar of brightly colored wooden mosaic pieces that they loved to smush around into their versions of Mars and Jupiter. Henry was Team Pluto. Charlie, the Lawyer, was not. "DATS NOTTA PLANET" he kept informing Henry in all caps. Charlie scooted over on his bottom, ready to fight. Ready to demolish. Henry hurriedly stuck his pudgy hand into the jar, trying heroically to keep Pluto relevant. He couldn't build fast enough because the jar opening was too narrow. Things were turning grim.

I walked over and looked down at both boys, both rotating in their own spheres of conflict, and then I bent down and, with a grand flourish, grabbed the jar and emptied the whole thing all over the floor with a loud clatter. The boys squealed. Look, Mom was being loud AND making a mess! They blinked up at me, the Founding Mother of Let's Not Dump It Out, and I think I just shrugged. It was raining outside. We needed the planets all over the dining room floor. And, we are Pluto-inclusive. Play resumed.

This is play. It can make a racket. Things spill. Bits might get lost or, worst of all, someone says it makes a mess or that it takes up too much time. We must persist at it with the loyalty of a toddler who loves Pluto.

The last time I felt afraid was just a few days ago. And there was really no reason why, except that it was 3:20 in the morning. Because menopause likes a pattern, my brain likes to zap itself awake at 3:20 in the morning a couple of times a week, just to make sure I'm still aware that the world is a horrible place. In that darkness that is neither morning nor night, the list unfurls before me, like one of those intros to a Star Wars movie:

THE BOYS ARE ON THEIR PHONES TOO MUCH

THE WASHING MACHINE IS LEAKING AGAIN

WHAT IF WE ALL LOST INTERNET POWER?

THE WEIRD BUMP ON MY KNEE IS CANCER.

SOMEDAY YOU'RE GONNA DIE.

Just once, I'd like my fears to be more tangible. Why can't I just be afraid of snakes? Or spiders? I could just be afraid of spiders. I'm not exactly enamored of a spider, honestly, but they don't freak me out much. If I find one in my house, I try to gently coax it out the door, where it can be creepy in the grass. Actually, now that I think of it, I do this because deep down I'm convinced that if I kill a spider, that spider's family is going to hold a meeting and plan a hit on me because they're all a part of the spider mafia. So, if I spy one, I talk real nice in a Bronx accent, and it goes into witness protection outside.

During my 3:20 a.m. appointments with dread, I try to breathe. I pray. My emotions are all at a level 10, and I need them to settle down. But it's now 3:27, and they still veer all around, from despair about a washing machine, then swooping over to anger about Brian's crazy work schedule. I pendulum back and forth and try to grab hold of the bedsheets for dear life.

Enter a scientist from California. Granted, this is a little crowded at 3:27 in our bedroom, but I need all the help I can get at this point, so I don't care. Dr.

Iris Mauss is the director of the Emotion and Emotion Regulation Lab at the University of California, Berkeley. She is a professor of social and personality psychology, and she has a lot to say about emotions.

She explains that one of the lab's main goals is helping people "reach goals for a good life." This sounds simple enough. We all want that. It's just that our stupid emotions keep messing it up, Mauss adds. "So often we think our emotions ARE us. But really, they are simply a response to a situation. The feeling? It's not the whole organism. We are experiences, behaviors, we are physiological . . . we are not *just* our feelings."

I told her about my recovery, how cravings and triggers are steeped in emotion, and how menopause had only exacerbated these tricky feelings. I talked and I talked, and Dr. Mauss listened and occasionally added a "hmm" to all my explanations. I'm not sure she signed up for this when she agreed to talk with me about recovery and emotions. I unload a list of feelings like I'm at the doctor's office. "And I have this weird spot on my knee!" I conclude. "It's scary!"

Ok, I don't tell her about my knee. I pull it together and decide to let her talk. Her voice is warm, softly accented with the clipped lilt of her German roots. I calm down. "Our work here is about helping people with managing that emotional piece," she says. "To not allow emotions to rule our lives and to live only at maximum intensity. That's not sustainable." I nod, picturing myself swinging from one emotional tree to the next like a super neurotic Tarzan. Then, I see myself collapse down to the earth, exhausted, empty, numb.

I tell her I think I must crave intensity. But also, I'm just so tired. "We all experience positive emotions, and negative ones too. One's life can absolutely include both the positive as well as the negative. There can be a richness there. They are not oppositional. They co-occur. They *need* to co-occur."

Last week, I attended the funeral of an 88-year-old grandmother with more than twenty-three grandkids. The pain of saying goodbye to her was paired with the joy of great-grandbabies, music, and happy memories. We accepted both things to honor Arlene: the tears and the laughter. Couldn't we practice this sort of acceptance in daily life? Could we practice funeral . . . living?

Mauss explains some techniques for regulating. "Be curious," she says. "Be aware. And be willing to do some work. You want to learn to regulate your emotions in accordance with your goals." She talks me through some techniques to help. Journaling helps with cognitive flexibility. Taking a pause helps us shake off the script.

Mauss also explained a technique that she said was her favorite. "It's kind of a lovely way to psychologically distance yourself from the situation. Use imagery to simply take yourself far away in time, physically, from the moment. For me, I just let myself float out into the Milky Way. We don't completely understand the science behind it yet, but I really like it because it's time, but it's like it's ten years later. This sort of reappraisal is abstract and so complicated, but our minds hook into it. It works really well."

And there it is. Iris is describing imaginative play. I don't do the Milky Way version because to me that seems rather terrifying (can I boop space?) but instead, I'm in Venice on a gondola, watching the sunset. For just a moment, I'm there and I'm breathing in the briny air and hearing opera. I trail my hand in the water. My brain sighs in Italian.

Dr. Iris Mauss is a mom, and I am comforted by this. Look! Scientists are moms too! She commiserates when I mention how I always wanted this to work with my children, how I feared their pain and their tears. "Kids are so highly emotional, and this collides with parents' urge for them to be happy. When my son was little, he would cry so much during that time, what do you call it? You know, the 'witching hour.'" I nod. Oh, I remember. My children are whining. My body and my brain long for wine. The tension of a five o'clock house.

Mauss continues. "Oh, how he cried. And I would think, 'There must be something I can do,' you know? To calm him down. But I just came to a point, probably because of exhaustion, really, where I realized 'I can't do anything. He's going to cry.' I just accepted it. I accepted that he is going to cry." She pauses for a moment, and I close my eyes. There is nothing but acceptance when it comes to parenting. To recovery. To life.

"And he would still fuss and cry, but my acceptance of it? It just transformed the whole situation. I would just be with him."

I would just be with him.

Perhaps that's what play does. I can just be with *me*. I dance around my living room before I start a run. I can't help it. My running playlist starts up with Florence and the Machine, and I start singing. My dogs are alarmed. This is my pre-run ritual. Then, at the end of every run, I reach up and pat myself on the back as I wheeze up the front porch steps. I do it every time. The neighbors might think I'm weird, but I'm not. I'm just playing.

I spot a house finch, one of my favorite little red birdies, chirping at me from a perch on the clematis at the end of the porch. He tilts his tiny head and scolds me. I tilt my head back and say, "Well, hello there, little guy," and right there I become a Bird Person. I download a bird app and start obsessing over this family of house finches. They are building a nest in the hanging fern. They probably just wish I would just leave them alone. I try to speak bird. I name them Louise and Vern in the Fern, and we all wait together for the eggs to hatch. I am convinced they secretly love me. My bird app picks up the song of something rare—a Fluffy Backed Tit-Babbler,[10] and I celebrate. I am middle-aged, therefore I bird. It becomes a thing, just me, my front porch, my post-run morning coffee, and my birds. It's play.

It's also ritual. Ritual gently grasps emotions and creates a holding place for them, organizing them into something comforting. My son draws a cross in the silty earth by home plate every time he comes up to bat. This is ritual. There's a pause. There's a bit more control. The brain benefits. Ritual calms us physiologically and mentally. Hopefully, there's a home run in there somewhere.

My morning conversations with Vern in the fern fend off anxiety. I didn't go into it with that in mind. I just wanted to make nice with Louise, Vern, and the kids. "Ritual" sounds so serious, so spiritual, it wafts of the much-overused word "wellness." It's just birds.[11] But it works. And I save it up, so that maybe the next time 3 a.m. beckons to me, my brain and I will be just a little bit stronger, a little bit readier to not play along with fear. There are games, and then there are wicked games, and I'm learning the difference.

Here is some further proof that all of us like a bit of play:

The World Extreme Ironing Championships: Brought to fame by the British documentary: *Extreme Ironing: Pressing for Victory*.[12] The first championship in Munich, Germany, had folks ironing on paddleboards in the river or while bicycling. One guy was ironing upside down, hanging off a climbing wall. Since that first fateful day, extreme ironing has shown up underwater, on cliffsides, and in marathons. As one who doesn't iron anymore because I wrote it out of my contract, I am especially enamored of the woman who sat up in a tree and yodeled while pressing a shirt. That's the way to do it.

Notes

1. My husband says "a stranger is just a friend I haven't met" and I asked him, what if the stranger is a serial killer. He told me that he never really thought of that before and that being married to me is so nice because I'm always willing to provide a different perspective. You're welcome, Brian.

2. This is what makes La Croix so *good*. I know there is something there, some deeply psychological reason that in my recovery I had to pick a drink that hurts a little going down as if each sip is making amends. I do love a drink with a good burn. Also, it's especially nice if you make a homemade strawberry syrup and add a sprig of mint. It's an amends drink, but make it fancy!

3. Also, do any of you remember thinking as a kid that you just could not wait to become a big, cool adult? What the frick, adulting.

4. This is a common phrase used in recovery, but I was first introduced to it in the film *28 Days*. No, this is not the zombie movie (although in a way it is). It's a movie where the main character, beautifully played by Sandra Bullock, is sent to rehab. It is one of my favorite movies about recovery. And I would know, because one thing addicts like to do when we stop drinking (or even prior) is watch and read every type of quit lit or film about people like us. So, it's movie night with buttered popcorn and therapy. Oh, and Viggo Mortensen. Highly recommend.

5. True story. College class. Beyond thrilling.

6. The merry-go-round is a super fun thing, until it's not. Much like drinking.

7. This, as my sons would say, is super cringe. Brian did mention that by the end of the week fewer people were responding to him and he wondered why.

8. I wish I had it when I was a kid and my parents decided to take us to the drive-in to see *Jaws* for whatever reason. I was afraid to take a bath for months after that experience.

9. 5063 US Highway 441 South
   Sylva, North Carolina 28779
   828.476.9376
   Call Harold if you want tickets. Open Daily!

10. Actual name of actual bird is not one I actually heard from my porch. I am using it as a stunt bird because the name is awesome.

11   Studies show that birding improves the brain's neuroplasticity. The "sorting" of birding, moving back and forth between objects of focus and their characteristics, strengthens focus and memory and puts us in a relaxed state of flow. Go forth and get yourself a little hat and some binoculars and get real immature about names like Fluffy Backed Tit-Babbler. Go birds!

12   This sport is not to be confused with Extreme Cello. Look it up.

Bibliography

1   **Play is biological:**
Wisseman, Nick (2021, November 17). Being Playful Is a Biological Imperative, Even for Adults. *Big Think*. https://bigthink.com/smart-skills/play-imperative-for-adults/.

2   **Information is simply a unit of the unexpected:**
Bernstein, Matthew N. (2020, June 13). What Is Information? (Foundations of Information Theory: Part 1). https://mbernste.github.io/posts/self_info/.

3   **A good surprise can shut down all of the brain's functions except the area devoted to reward:**
Hughes, Melissa (2023, March 31). The Science of Surprise. *Neuro Nugget*. https://www.melissahughes.rocks/post/the-science-of-surprise#:~:text=Not%20only%20do%20you%20get.

4   **The nucleus accumbens, the reward area of the brain that lights up due to surprise, is also where addicted cravings are generated:**
UK-Rehab (n.d.). Nucleus-Accumbens | Addiction Psychology | UK Rehab. Accessed July 7, 2024. https://www.uk-rehab.com/addiction-psychology/nucleus-accumbens/#:~:text=.

5   **Fred Rogers made a song for this very thing, aptly titled *You Can Never Go Down the Drain:***
King, Maxwell (2018, June 8). Mr. Rogers's Simple Set of Rules for Talking to Kids. *The Atlantic*. https://www.theatlantic.com/family/archive/2018/06/mr-rogers-neighborhood-talking-to-kids/562352/.

6   **As we age, we don't have as many "new" images to process, so time works more quickly:**
Livni, Ephrat (2019, January 8). Physics Explains Why Time Passes Faster as You Age. *Quartz*. https://qz.com/1516804/physics-explains-why-time-passes-faster-as-you-age#:~:text=They%20flow%20at%20varying%20rates.

7   **The brain is benefited:**
Baron, Jessica (2022, June 21). How Rituals Rewire Your Brain. *Spirituality+Health*. https://www.spiritualityhealth.com/how-rituals-rewire-your-brain.

8   **The World Extreme Ironing Championships:**
Britclip. (2019, June 19). "The World Extreme Ironing Championships." https://www.youtube.com/watch?v=7fd6NBQ8ego.

18

Big Time Dessert

I think the only way we get out of this life alive is if we're willing to be curious about ourselves. Even then, the chances are slim.

For a long time, I was never able to do battle with More. I have never been an assertive person. I never wanted to hurt alcohol's feelings, and so I just succumbed. More wine. More vodka. Then all that got kicked out, but More chocolate sidled up. More exercise did too. More futile addiction to certainty, so I could feel sated and not ever afraid. I did all this so I would never have to look Less in the eye.

Dessert is abundance. But it's also about inviting Less to the table. I know who I am now. I've lived with myself long enough to figure myself out. Oh, and also? I give myself permission to be afraid. Fear and Less are often the same. I am remarkably able to feel fear and strength at the same time. I hold tight to some things, and I scatter the rest. It's all part of the sweetness of the lemon in the pie.

When all of this started for me, with the process addictions rearing their stubborn heads and the menopause and mental health diagnosis, I was in the middle of living my dream. I was an author on a book tour. I had hotel rooms and an itinerary, and a suitcase with wheels. This is what I have always wanted since I was a little girl: to be an author.

But along with all those accomplishments came loneliness and fear. They were my two hotel bedfellows. I could have allowed that space to be where I gave up. It would have been sort of easy, especially after a sparsely attended book signing where one woman came in and grabbed a chair, and then volunteered after my talk, "I'm just here because I needed to sit down." That lady is kind of my hero, both for her utter disregard for social cues and for her ability to humble me whenever I start to think I am a big deal.

But hey, I didn't give up. This book is hopefully something that helps show others what it's like to stay on the path of sobriety or just life-ing. Women "of a certain age" have a lot to contend with, in my opinion. We do battle. It's exhausting.

But here's something else that happened on that book tour. My final hotel had also booked a large Indian wedding. The morning that I was heading home, I rolled into the elevator, and right as the doors were closing, I heard "Hold! Please!" in a lilting voice. Then, I was accosted by color. Six women, bedecked in shimmering sarees and jewels and thick perfume, stepped into the small space. Their bracelets and earrings softly jingled as they moved, and their voices were like music. It was like riding in an elevator with a bunch of tropical birds. One woman kept asking for help with her earrings, which were caught in her long hair. There was giggling. We rode down, and as the doors slid open, I blurted out, "You all look so pretty." They responded with more smiles and quiet "Thank yous" and then fluttered away. I kept spotting them as I was checking out, popping up in a brilliant wash of chartreuse or gold or pink, floating out the front doors to meet another colorful contingent, all chirping excitedly, or sitting incongruously next to a business guy in Dockers reading his phone.

Then, there were the babies on the plane. I was seated near the back, and one baby was in the seat in front of me. He kept crawling up on his mom's shoulder, as tall as he could, and looking out over all the heads before him. Then, he crowed. A beat later, a second baby, near the front, crowed back. There was a third baby somewhere who also joined in. They were talking to each other. Passengers started laughing as these three had their own baby meetup while we headed for the runway. It was lovely.

I paid attention. I stored these moments up, writing them down in a little notebook I have for such occasions. I kept watching.

I had a layover in Chicago and went hunting for the Nuts on Clark stand. As I waited in line, checking my phone to make sure I had the time, I sighed. I was tired. I wanted to get home.

The lady who waited on me had a strong Slavic accent, and I leaned in to ask her to repeat herself when she spoke to me. "Sorry, I don't have the best ears. What did you say?"

She repeated, "I say, how was your day today?"

I smiled. "Good. Tired. Ready to get home."

She eyed me from under her cap, her blond hair tucked in wayward tufts around her face. She looked like a mom. And then she sealed that deal by saying the most mom thing ever: "You breathe. You must take deep breath in. Ok? It's all going to be good soon!" Her smile was as wide as the sky. I felt tears hitting my eyelids as I nodded. "Deep breath, momma.[1] Home soon, right?" and she handed me a warm paper bag of almond caramel corn. "This will help."

"Deep breath." I nodded.

"I work here a long time. Everybody just wants to get home." She smiled even wider. She had a gap between her teeth, and her eyes crinkled. I wanted to hug her.

We all just want to get home, back to the center of things.

These little moments, these holy spaces, they bolster me. I am propped up in my weariness by stories and the essential goodness of people. Stories heal. When you tell someone a story, the listener and the speaker both experience a "lining up" of neural activity; putting each other, literally, on the same brain wave. It's like the brain loves listening to a story so much it sighs and leans forward, clasping hands with the storyteller's brain. That's communication at its finest. It's how I found my way through early recovery. It's how I find peace when I'm unpeaceful.

It's how this book came to be.

In August of 2023, Hurricane Idalia landed in the Big Bend area of Florida. Idalia was a category 4 hurricane, the third-largest hurricane that area has ever known, creating wreckage that covered over half of the state. The devastation was complete.

And then, about a year later, people started to spot the flamingos.

The iconic bird has long been associated with Florida, but due to the plume trade and urbanization, they had all but disappeared. There were very few wild flamingos left in the state despite the massive marketing and iconography (*Miami Vice*, anyone?) telling us otherwise.

But after Idalia, people kept seeing them. Sightings were happening all over the shorelines, with avid bird watchers traveling and excitedly spying whole improbable pink clumps of them, just standing around looking gorgeous. Nobody was exactly sure why this was happening; scientists said they probably blew in. The numbers kept increasing. More accounts came in. People were counting more birds in a week than had been reported since the early 1900s.

They had returned. It took wreckage and destruction, but here they are. Glossy pink, fabulous feathery miracles. Right back in their original home.

And they are beautiful.

Note

1 How did she know?

Bibliography

1 **... the listener and the speaker both experience a "lining up" neural activity:**
Suzuki, Wendy A., Mónica I. Feliú-Mójer, Uri Hasson, Rachel Yehuda, and Jean Mary Zarate (2018). Dialogues: The Science and Power of Storytelling. *The Journal of Neuroscience* 38 (44): 9468–70. https://doi.org/10.1523/jneurosci.1942-18.2018.

2 **... people started to spot the flamingos:**
Rozsa, Lori (2024, May 26). How Florida Is Getting Its Pink Back." *Washington Post*. https://www.washingtonpost.com/nation/interactive/2024/florida-flamingo-idalia-hurricane-everglades/.

Epilogue
Hashtag Blessed

One of the first recovery meetings I ever attended made me mad. Everyone in the room was settled. Nobody shifted around or seemed uncomfortable. They all knew each other, and no one was talking to me, and I felt weird. Or weirder, as I had just given up the one thing that seemed to be my anti-weird leveling agent for over twenty years.

I shifted in my seat again, and it stuck to the back of my thighs. It was hot outside. A small oscillating fan stirred the soupy air in the room. The coffee pot in the corner of the room smelled of shellac. I had been sober for a couple of weeks, and this was starting to seem like a horrible decision. Feelings kept zinging around in me, spurting out with no warning, and it's really difficult to get mad at *everything* when you're not mad at *everything*. You're mad, very specifically, at certain things, but *everything* will have to suffice right now because you're just starting on this journey, and your brain can't get organized. Also, I hated that it was even a journey. Couldn't it just be quick, like a one-month retreat? Maybe with a lot of massages and some water with cucumber slices floating in it?

We were going around the room and talking. This one guy who looked like a roadie for Lynyrd Skynyrd said, "I'm a grateful alcoholic. My name is Phil," and he started in on how blessed he was about being an addict in the first place, how his addiction had been a gift to him. He spoke about strength and joy and blah blah blah, and I kept glitching on that word "blessed."

I mean, it's hard to be blessed when you're building a prison.

When I started to understand addiction a little better, I forgave Phil for annoying me at that meeting, which was really nice of me. I am pretty sure Phil has no idea who I am, but I still think about him. He smiled a lot when he spoke, and he always looked peaceful.

And now I say the same thing. I say that I am a grateful alcoholic. I stole his words. Addicts do that. We often hear the stories of others, chew on them, and then they become our own. And nobody cares that we steal those words because we are not at all worried about plagiarism in recovery circles.

Middle-aged white women have thrown the word "blessed" around so much. Especially us Christian folk. We kinda ruined it. Sorry. We started with the hashtag and the wooden signs in our living rooms and felt hats with wide brims, and from there, we just got annoying. Sorry. Sorry about that.

So, maybe I'll just use this word: *Strong*.

Everybody does strong differently. My version has me reckoning with salads, practicing acceptance, and squaring up with grace. We are all so very different. We all face addiction with different paths ahead. This book is my own wonky journey. I hope it helps someone. If all else fails, it does have a fabulous lemon pie recipe.

I went on a long run this morning, and I did not feel strong. About two blocks in, my main thoughts were "Do not fall down," and "This hurts." Some runs are like that. I kept going. When I was done, I patted myself on the shoulder, gasped up the stairs, and felt better. It's a morning exchange. Prior to the run, my thoughts say: *A run will hurt. Just stay home.* But it's going to hurt either way. The run will hurt. But my brain will hurt if I *don't* run. So, it's a choice. When I chose to walk away from alcohol, it hurt. Sobriety hurts. It's hard. But so did my soured, addicted soul. So, which hurt do I choose? It was exchanging bad suffering for good suffering. That's why Phil ticked me off. And that's why I still remember him.

We are all addicted to something. And, as I get older, I realize I just wanted the kind of pain in my life that is still interesting. There's the pain of learning, change, growth, and persistence, and that's the hurt that's worth it.

A Recipe for Lemon Pie

A Recipe for Lemon Pie That Will Make You Hurt a Little, It's So Good

Ingredients

1 cup sugar

¼ cup corn starch

1 cup of lemon juice from real actual lemons.

3 egg yolks, beaten

Pinch salt

Peel of one lemon—grated

⅓ cup of cold water (might use a bit more)

A knob of butter ('Knob' is the right term. Grandmas know).

9-inch pie crust—baked. I use store-bought even though it's not the best. Making a homemade pie crust is no longer something I want to do with my life.

Whipped cream. Ok, many will think this pie should have a meringue topping, and I think it did originally. I don't like meringue. So, I made homemade whipped cream, which is superior in every way.

To make homemade whipped cream: Chill your bowl in the freezer for five minutes. Then, pour in one of those smaller containers of heavy whipping cream, a pinch of salt, a dollop of vanilla, and a ½ cup of powdered sugar. Put on your stand mixer if you have one and let 'er rip until it looks like whipped cream. Don't overdo it, or you'll end up with very sweet butter, which honestly isn't so bad either. Great on Graham crackers. Or so I've heard.

If you want: Use Cool Whip. It's also very tasty.

Instructions

Combine one cup of sugar and cornstarch in a medium saucepan. Gradually stir in lemon juice and water until smooth. Stir in egg yolks and salt.

Bring to a gentle plopping boil over medium heat, stirring constantly, and boil for 1 minute. Remove from heat. Stir in lemon peel and butter.

Spoon hot filling into the pie crust. Try not to sample the hot filling because you will burn your fingers, or so I have heard. Let the pie sit out for a bit until you can put it on a tray and chill it in the fridge for an hour. Artistically smear on the whipped cream. Let it chill for a few more hours and then devour.

Index

abstinence 64
acceptance 251
addiction 10, 50, 52, 144
addictive behaviors 19, 244
addictive cravings 244
alcohol 77
alcoholics 17, 90
    grade-A alcoholic 36
alcoholism 19, 76, 84, 103
amygdala 133, 149
anti-aging 167
anxiety 50, 72, 75, 139
Apostrophe Protection Society 204
appetizers 126
audiologist 117–18

bad brain 102
behavioral addictions 65
Big-C creativity 227
book tour 9–10
boredom 201–2
Bottled 57

caregiver burnout 60
Cave Syndrome 93
citizen scientists 223
clinical depression 121–2
codependency 85, 87, 89, 91
cognitive distortions 61
Cold-turkey alcohol 35
Continued forward movement (CFM) 230–2

control and perfectionism 139
Covid tests 160
creative mortification 229
creativity 224, 228

depression 84, 92, 102, 119
diabetes 212
dissociative disorder 78
donuts 57–9, 61–2
double pandemic 33
Dull Women's Club 244

eating disorder 84
Elevenses 13
Emotion Regulation Lab 250
endorphins 241
estrogen 87
exposure therapy 148

fair to poor 24
fear 247
forgiveness 179, 190, 192

global pandemic 27–9
    alcohol consumption 38–40
    alcoholism 34–7
guilt 85

Hawaii Space Exploration Analog and Simulation (HI-SEAS) 204
hibernation 9
hormonal anxiety 141

hormone replacement therapy 72
hospitalization 121
How to Be Perfect Like Me 9, 13, 162

imposter syndrome 10
impulsivity 218
inferior parietal cortex 164
Invisible Women Syndrome 166
Iowa Writers Workshop 12
isolation 25–7, 37
    executive function in brain 32–3
    social 33–4, 37
isolation gauge 28

League of Good Women 111
lemon pie 60
limbic system 61
lizard brain 61
long-term recovery 242

menopausal fatigue 141
menopause 69–71, 77, 85, 90
    hormone fluctuations 86
midlife crisis 200
moderation 64
motion-sickness progression 11

NASA scientists 204
negativity bias 15
neuroses 101
nucleus accumbens 244

object permanence 202

Pavlovian alcoholic 126
pelvic exam 70
pendulum behavior 147
perfectionism 85
playfulness 242
postpartum depression 71, 161
prefrontal cortex 56, 173
premenopausal 70, 72, 102
process addictions 87, 148, 179, 255
progesterone 87

realistic optimism 113–14
Repeated Negative Thinking (RNT) 17
risky behavior 159

self-forgiveness 188–9
Shallow Forgiveness 133
shame 144–5, 183
Shitty Forgiveness 133
sober foreverness 198
sobriety 7, 49, 66, 103, 148, 159
    marriage 103–5
        pros and cons 105–6
social anxiety 84
stress 75, 79, 127, 129, 131
sugar 50, 53–4, 131
suicidal ideation 121

teenage depression 151
temporal cortex 173
tinnitus 116
trigger 147

Xanax 79, 83

About the Author

Dana Bowman is the author of two other memoirs, *Bottled, A Mom's Guide to Early Recovery,* and *How to Be Perfect Like Me,* both published by Central Recovery Press. *Bottled* was selected as a Kansas Notable Book in 2018.

A TEDx speaker, writer for *Psychology Today,* and occasional stand-up comedian, she shares about beating shame, kicking addictions, and how going gray changed her life. Dana was a high school English teacher for over twenty years and now teaches writing and digital media at Bethany College in Lindsborg, Kansas. She also works at her happy place, her small-town library, in the afternoons. There, she gets to wear weird clothes and is in charge of children's programming. She is a tired mom of two teenage boys and hopes one day that the sports schedule will slow down so she can go on a date with her husband. One can dream.

Dana has collected numerous awards for her humorous writing, and she earned the moniker of "The Erma Bombeck of alcoholics" from her first publisher, a descriptor she is very proud to carry. Her goal is to provide hope, along with a good laugh and a good story, to help heal the addict within all of us.

You can connect with her on all the socials (even TikTok because she is cool) at @thedanabow, or over at her website: danabowmancreative.com